FAMINE AND DISEASE IN IRELAND

VOLUME V

FAMINE AND DISEASE IN IRELAND

Volume V

Edited by Leslie A. Clarkson and E. Margaret Crawford

Routledge
Taylor & Francis Group
LONDON AND NEW YORK

First published 2005 by Pickering & Chatto (Publishers) Limited

2 Park Square, Milton Park, Abingdon, Oxon OX14 4RN
711 Third Avenue, New York, NY 10017, USA

Routledge is an imprint of the Taylor & Francis Group, an informa business

First issued in paperback 2017

BRITISH LIBRARY CATALOGUING IN PUBLICATION DATA
Famine and disease in Ireland
1. Famines – Ireland – History – 19th century 2. Famines – Ireland – History – 18th century 3. Public health – Ireland – History – 19th century 4. Public health – Ireland – History – 18th century 5. Nutritionally induced diseases – Ireland – History – 19th century 6. Nutritionally induced diseases – Ireland – History – 18th century 7. Ireland – Social conditions – 19th century 8. Ireland – Social conditions – 18th century 9. Ireland – History – Famine, 1845–1852 10. Ireland – History – 18th century
I. Clarkson, Leslie A. II. Crawford, E. Margaret
363.8'09415'09034

LIBRARY OF CONGRESS CATALOGING-IN-PUBLICATION DATA
A catalogue record for this title is available from the Library of Congress.

ISBN-13: 978-1-1387-5336-5 (hbk)
ISBN-13: 978-1-138-11146-2 (pbk)
ISBN-13: 978-1-85196-791-9 (set)

CONTENTS

CHRONOLOGY

Jonathan Swift (1667–1745)

[*Note*: For a comprehensive chronology of Swift see the *Oxford Dictionary of National Biography* (*ODNB*) (Oxford: Oxford University Press, 2004)]

1667	Born Dublin, 30 November, second child of Jonathan Swift (1640–67) and Abigail Erick (1640–1710).
1668	Sent to England where he stays for three years.
*c.*1673–81	Attended Kilkenny College.
1682	April, enters Trinity College, Dublin.
1689	Leaves Ireland for England and enters the service of Sir William Temple.
1690–4	Divides his time between England and Ireland.
1694	Ordained in Dublin and appointed curate to Kilroot, Co. Antrim, but spends much of his time in England.
1699	Returns to Dublin and becomes Chaplain to the Earl of Berkeley. Divides his time between Dublin and England and begins his publishing career.
1714	Appointed Dean of St Patrick's, Dublin.
1720	Begins publishing pamphlets on Irish affairs including, in 1724, the *Drapier's Letters*.
1726	Publishes *Gulliver's Travels*.
1727–8	Publishes *A Short View*.
1729	Publishes *A Modest Proposal*.
1742	Declared 'of unsound mind'.
1745	Dies in Dublin, October 19.

John Rutty (1698–1775)

1698	Born Melksham, Wiltshire, 25 December, younger son of John and Ester Rutty, Quakers.

1723	Graduates Medical Doctor (MD) from the University of Leiden.
1724	Settles in Dublin.
1729	Enrols as a Licentiate Fellow of the King and Queen's College of Physicians in Ireland.
1744	A founder member of the Physico-Historical Society.
1751	Publishes *A History of the Rise and Progress of the People called Quakers in Ireland.*
1757	Publishes *A Methodical Synopsis of Mineral Waters.*
1762	Publishes *The Analysis of Milk.*
1770	Publishes *A Chronological History of the Weather and Seasons, and of the Prevailing Diseases in Dublin: with the Various Periods, Successions, and Revolutions, during the Space of Forty Years ...*
1772	Publishes *An Essay towards a Natural History of the County of Dublin.*
1775	Publishes *Materia medica antiqua et nova.*
1775	Dies in Dublin, 27 April.
1776	*A Spiritual Diary and Soliloquies* (two volumes) published posthumously.

William Harty (1781–1854)

1781	Born in Kilkenny, son of Timothy Harty, gentleman.
1797	Enters Trinity College, Dublin. Graduates Bachelor of Arts (BA) in 1801, Bachelor of Medicine (MB) in 1804, Medical Doctor (MD) in 1830.
1818	Licentiate of the King and Queen's College of Physicians in Ireland: Fellow 1824; Censor (i.e. Examiner) 1830; Honorary Fellow 1833.
1818	Founder member of the Association for the Suppression of Street-Begging in Dublin.
1820s–	Physician to the Poor Sick Institution, the King's Hospital and the Dublin prisons.
1820	Publishes *Historic Sketch of the Causes, Extent, and Mortality of Contagious Fever, Epidemic in Ireland in 1741, and during 1817, 1818, and 1819*
*c.*1820	Becomes the owner of Finglas House, a private lunatic asylum.

1851 Sued for assault by Henry William Mathew, Harty's natural son, whom Harty had committed as a lunatic to the asylum. Mathew was awarded £1,000 damages.

1854 Dies Ballickmoyler, Queen's County, 30 March.

Swift (1727–8)
A Short View of the State of Ireland

A Short View of the State of Ireland [By Jonathan Swift] (Dublin: S. Harding, 1727–8).

A Short View was written at the end of 1727. It was published anonymously early the following year, but its author was Jonathan Swift, the Dean of St Patrick's Dublin. Had there been any doubt about its authorship, the reference to Lord Chief Justice Whitshed, an old judicial foe of Swift's, would have speedily dispelled it. The pamphlet was reprinted in the *Intelligencer,* a weekly paper edited by Swift and Thomas Sheridan probably in November 1728, where it was attributed to the 'Drapier', the pseudonym of Swift.

In 1728 Archbishop Boulter of Dublin wrote that 'the dearness of corn was such that thousands of families quitted their habitations to seek bread elsewhere, and many hundreds perished'.[1] But the *Short View* was only indirectly concerned with famine. Instead Swift concentrated on what he regarded as more fundamental weaknesses in society, including crippling restrictions on Irish trade and industry, the spread of grazing at the expense of arable farming, rent remittances to landlords living in England, and the taste among the wealthy minority for foreign imports at the expense of home manufactures.

Within a few days of publishing *A Short View* Swift received a pamphlet from an anonymous author entitled *The Memorial of the Poor Inhabitants, Tradesmen, and Labourers of the Kingdom of Ireland.*[2] It argued that in 1727 'there was a very great Scarcity of Bread Corn' and that but for imports the poor 'would have perished for want of Bread'. So bad were the shortages that people 'were forced ... to fall too soon upon their early Corn and Potatoes'. Even so, famine was widespread among the poor, which 'has often been the Occasion of Pestilential and contagious Distempers, whereby the Rich have become sharers in the general Calamity....' The

1. Quoted in L.A. Clarkson and E. Margaret Crawford, *Feast and Famine: A History of Food and Nutrition in Ireland 1500–1920* (Oxford: Oxford University Press, 2001), p. 125.

2. The author was John Browne who was known to Swift for his part in the controversy over Wood's halfpennies. The pamphlet is printed in Herbert Davies (ed.), *Jonathan Swift, Irish Tracts 1728–1733* (Oxford: Oxford University Press, 1955), pp. 303–5.

author argued that premiums should be offered to importers of corn, paid for by a tax on luxury imports.

Swift responded in a pamphlet of his own.[1] In it he reiterated the arguments of *A Short View*. The difficulties of the 1720s arose not from temporary difficulties but from long-term causes, particularly the rapacious behaviour of graziers and the neglect of arable farming. The plan to tax luxuries he dismissed as 'visionary' because it would simply depress consumption and so revenues would fall. In any case, if corn were imported the poor could not afford to buy it. He subsequently summarized his position in a letter to Alexander Pope in August 1729: 'As to this country, there have been three terrible years' dearth of corn, and every place strewed with beggars; but dearths are common in better climates, and our evils here lie much deeper.'[2]

The exchange between Swift and his correspondent foreshadowed an issue raised by modern students of famine. As Professor Arnold has pointed out famine 'is both event and structure'.[3] That is to say, there are short-term causes of famine. In 1727–9 these were a series of bad seasons that ruined the corn; in 1740–1 it was the great frost; in 1845–9 it was the potato blight. But such events would have been less catastrophic had the structure of society been more robust. According to Swift the difficulties of 1727–9 were compounded by the extension of grazing during the previous decades; he might also have pointed to the growth of population since the beginning of the century, which added perhaps ten per cent (a quarter of a million people) to the total. The penetrating frost of 1740–1 that turned the potatoes into mush might have been less disastrous had they not become so important as items of diet, although the greater hardship was suffered in the cities where the poor could not afford to buy corn. And the Great Famine a century later would have been less great had three million people not been living almost exclusively on potatoes and buttermilk.

When *A Short View* was republished in the *Intelligencer* Thomas Sheridan recommended that every householder should frame every page and hang them in every chamber of their houses. This seems a little extreme today. But it is worth reading by scholars of famines in Ireland as a trenchant if not wholly objective analysis of the long-term problems underlying the short-term crisis of the late 1720s.

1. 'An Answer to a Paper called a Memorial ...' in Davies, *Jonathan Swift. Irish Tracts*, pp. 10–25.

2. Quoted in Davies, *Jonathan Swift, Irish Tracts*, p. xix.

3. David Arnold, *Famine; Social Crisis and Historical Change* (Oxford: B. Blackwell, 1988), p. 6.

A
Short VIEW
OF THE
STATE
OF
IRELAND.

DUBLIN:
Printed by *S. HARDING*, next Door to the *Crown* in *Copper-Alley*, 1727-8.

[1]

A

Short View, &c.

I Am assured that it hath for some time been practised as a method of making Men's Court, when they are asked about the Rate of Lands, the Abilities of Tenants, the State of Trade and Manufacture in this Kingdom, and how their Rents are payed; to Answer, That in their Neighbourhood all things are in a flourishing Condition, the Rent and Purchase of Land every Day encreasing. And if a Gentleman happens to be a little more sincere in his Representations, besides being looked on as not well affected, he is sure to have a Dozen Contradictors

dictors at his Elbow. I think it is no manner of Secret why these Questions are so cordially asked, or so obligingly Answered.

But since with Regard to the Affairs of this Kingdom, I have been using all Endeavours to subdue my Indignation, to which indeed I am not provoked by any Personal Interest, being not the Owner of one Spot of Ground in the whole *Island*, I shall only enumerate by Rules generally known, and never Contradicted, what are the true Causes of any Countries flourishing and growing Rich, and then examine what Effects arise from those Causes in the Kingdom of *Ireland*.

The first Cause of a Kingdom's thriving is the Fruitfulness of the Soyl, to produce the Necessaries and Conveniencies of Life, not only sufficient for the Inhabitants, but for Exportation into other Countries.

The Second, is the Industry of the People in Working up all their Native Commodities to the last degree of Manufacture.

The Third, is the Conveniency of safe Ports and Havens, to Carry out their own Goods, as much manufactured, and bring in those of others, as little manufactured as the Nature of mutual Commerce will allow.

The Fourth, is, That the Natives should as much as possible, Export and Import their Goods in Vessels of their own Timber, made in their own Country. The

The Fifth, is the Liberty of a free Trade in all Foreign Countries, which will permit them, except to thofe who are in War with their own Prince or State.

The Sixth, is, by being Governed only by Laws made with their own Confent, for otherwife they are not a free People. And therefore all Appeals for Juftice, or Applications, for Favour or Preferment to another Country, are fo many grievous Impoverifhments.

The Seventh, is, by Improvement of Land, encouragement of Agriculture, and thereby encreafing the Number of their People, without which any Country, however Bleffed by Nature, muft continue Poor.

The Eighth, is the Refidence of the Princes, or Chief Adminiftrators of the Civil Power.

The Ninth, is the Concourfe of Foreigners, for Education, Curiofity or Pleafure, or as to a general Mart of Trade.

The Tenth, is by difpofing all Offices of Honour, Profit or Truft, only to the Natives, or at leaft with very few Exceptions, where Strangers have long Inhabited the Country, and are fuppofed to Underftand, and regard the Intereft of it as their own.

The Eleventh is, when the Rents of Lands, and Profits of Employments are fpent in the Country which produced them, and not in in another, the former of which will certainly happen, where the Love of our Native Country prevails.

The Twelfth, is by the publick Revenues being all Spent and Employed at Home, except on the Occasions of a Foreign War.

The Thirteenth, is, where the People are not obliged, unless they find it for their own Interest, or Conveniency, to receive any Monies, except of their own Coynage by a publick Mint, after the manner of all Civilized Nations.

The Fourteenth, is a Disposition of a People of a Country to wear their own Manufactures, and Import as few Incitements to Luxury, either in Cloaths, Furniture, Food or Drink, as they possibly can live conveniently without.

There are many other Causes of a Nation's thriving, which I cannot at present recollect, but without Advantage from at least some of these; after turning my Thoughts a long time, I am not able to discover from whence our Wealth proceeds, and therefore would gladly be better informed. In the mean time, I will here examine what share falls to *Ireland* of these Causes, or of the Effects and Consequences.

It is not my Intention to complain, but barely to relate Facts, and the matter is not

of

of ſmall Importance. For it is allowed, that a Man who lives in a Solitary Houſe far from help, is not Wiſe in endeavouring to acquire in the Neighbourhood, the Reputation of being Rich, becauſe thoſe who come for Gold, will go off with Pewter and Braſs, rather than return empty; and in the common Practice of the World, thoſe who poſſeſs moſt Wealth, make the leaſt Parade, which they leave to others, who have nothing elſe to bear them out, in ſhewing their Faces on the *Exchange.*

As to the firſt Cauſe of a Nation's Riches, being the Fertility of the Soyl, as well as Temperature of Clymate we have no Reaſon to complain; for although the Quantity of unprofitable Land in this Kingdom, reckoning Bog, and Rock, and barren Mountain, be double in Proportion to what it is in *England*, yet the Native Productions which both Kingdoms deal in, are very near on equality in point of Goodneſs, and might with the ſame Encouragement be as well manufactured, I except Mines and Minerals, in ſome of which however we are only defective in point of Skill and Induſtry.

In the Second, which is the Induſtry of the People, our misfortune is not altogether owing to our own Fault, but to a million of Diſcouragements.

The

The conveniency of Ports and Havens which Nature bestowed us so liberally is of no more use to us, than a beautiful Prospect to a Man shut up in a Dungeon.

As to Shipping of it's own, this Kingdom is so utterly unprovided, that of all the excellent Timber cut down within these fifty or sixty Years, it can hardly be said that the Nation hath received the Benefit of one valuable House to dwell in, or one Ship to Trade with.

Ireland is the only Kingdom I ever heard or read of, either in ancient or modern Story, which was denyed the Liberty of exporting then native Commodities and Manufactures wherever they pleased, except to Countries at War with their own Prince or State, yet this by the Superiority of meer Power is refused us in the most momentous parts of Commerce, besides an Act of Navigation to which we never consented, pinned down upon us, and rigorously executed, and a thousand other unexampled Circumstances as grievous as they are invidious to mention. To go unto the Rest.

It is too well known that we are forced to obey some Laws we never consented to, which is a Condition I must not call by it's true unconverted Name for fear of my *L—C— J—W—*'s Ghost with his *LIBERTAS ET NATALE*

NATALE SOLUM, written as a Motto on his Coach, as it ſtood at the Door of the Court, while he was Perjuring himſelf to betray both. Thus, we are in the Condition of Patients who have Phyſick ſent them by Doctors at a Diſtance, Strangers to their Conſtitution, and the nature of their Diſeaſe: And thus, we are forced to pay five hundred *per Cent* to divide our Properties, in all which we have likewiſe the Honour to be diſtinguiſhed from the whole Race of Mankind.

As to improvement of Land, thoſe few who attempt that or Planting, through Covetouſneſs or want of Skill, generally leave things worſe than they were, neither ſucceeding in Trees nor Hedges, and by running into the fancy of Grazing after the manner of the *Scythians*, are every Day depopulating the Country.

We are ſo far from having a King to reſide among us, that even the Viceroy is generally abſent four Fifths of his time in the Government.

No Strangers from other Countries make this a part of their Travels, where they can expect to ſee nothing but Scenes of Miſery and Deſolation.

Thoſe who have the Misfortune to be born here, have the leaſt Title to any conſiderable Employment, to which they are ſeldom preferred, but upon a Political Conſideration.

One

[10]

One third part of the Rents of *Ireland* is ſpent in *England*, which with the Profit of Employments, Penſions, Appeals, Journeys of Pleaſure or Health, Education at the *Inns* of Court, and both Univerſities, Remittances at Pleaſure, the Pay of all Superior Officers in the Army and other Incidents, will amount to a full half of the Income of the whole Kingdom, all clear profit to *England*.

We are denyed the Liberty of Coining Gold, Silver, or even Copper. In the Iſle of *Man*, they Coin their own Silver, every petty Prince, Vaſſal to the *Emperor* can Coin what Money he pleaſeth. And in this as in moſt of the Articles already mentioned, we are an exception to all other States or Monarchies that were ever known in the World.

As to the laſt, or Fourteenth Article, we take ſpecial Care to Act diametrically contrary to it in the whole Courſe of our Lives. Both Sexes, but eſpecially the Women deſpiſe and abhor to wear any of their own Manufactures, even thoſe which are better made than in other Countries, particularly a ſort of Silk Plad, through which the Workmen are forced to run a ſort of Gold-thread that it may paſs for *Indian*. Even Ale and Potatoes in great quantity are Imported from *England* as well as Corn, and our foreign Trade is little more than Importation of *French* Wine, for which I am told we pay ready Money.

Now

Now if all this be true, upon which I could eaſily enlarge, I would be glad to know by what ſecret method it is that we grow a Rich and Flouriſhing People, without Liberty, Trade, Manufactures, Inhabitants, Money, or the privilege of Coining; without Induſtry, Labour or Improvement of Lands, and with more than half of the Rent and Profits of the whole *Kingdom*, Annually exported, for which we receive not a ſingle Farthing: And to make up all this, nothing worth mentioning, except the Linnen of the *North* a Trade caſual corrupted and at Mercy, and ſome Butter from *Cork*. If we do flouriſh, it muſt be againſt every Law of Nature and Reaſon, like the Thorn at *Glaſſenbury*, that bloſſoms in the midſt of Winter.

Let the worthy *C——rs* who come from *England* ride round the Kingdom, and obſerve the face of Nature, or the faces of the Natives, the Improvement of the Land, the thriving numerous Plantations, the noble Woods, the abundance and vicinity of Country-Seats, the commodious Farmers-Houſes and Barns, the Towns and Villages, where every body is buſy and thriving with all kind of Manufactures, the Shops full of Goods wrought to Perfection, and filled with Cuſtomers, the comfortable Dyet and Dreſs, and Dwellings of the People, the vaſt Numbers of Ships in our

Harbours

Harbours and Docks, and Shipwrights in our Seaport-Towns. The Roads crouded with Carryers laden with rich Manufactures, the perpetual Concourse to and fro of pompous Equipages.

With what Envy and Admiration would these Gentlemen return from so delightful a Progress? What glorious Reports would they make when they went back to *England*?

But my Heart is too heavy to continue this Journey longer, for it is manifest that whatever Stranger took such a Journey, would be apt to think himself travelling in *Lapland* or *Island*, rather than in a Country so favoured by Nature as Ours, both in Fruitfulness of Soyl, and Temperature of Climate. The miserable Dress, and Dyet, and Dwelling of the People. The general Desolation in most parts of the Kingdom. The old Seats of the Nobility and Gentry all in Ruins, and no new Ones in their stead. The Families of Farmers who pay great Rents, living in Filth and Nastiness upon Butter-milk and Potatoes, without a Shoe or Stocking to their Feet, or a House so convenient as an *English* Hog-sty to receive them. These indeed may be comfortable sights to an *English* Spectator, who comes for a short time only *to learn the Language*, and returns back to his own Country,

Country, whither he finds all our Wealth transmitted.

Nostrâ miseriâ magnus es.

There is not one Argument used to prove the Riches of *Ireland*, which is not a logical Demonstration of it's Poverty. The Rise of our Rents is squeesed out of the very Blood and Vitals, and Cloaths, and Dwellings of the Tenants who live worse than *English* Beggars. The lowness of Interest in all other Countries a sign of Wealth is in us a proof of misery, there being no Trade to employ any Borrower. Hence alone comes the Dearness of Land, since the Savers have no other way to lay out their Money. Hence the Dearness of Necessaries for Life, because the Tenants cannot afford to pay such extravagant Rates for Land (which they must take, or go a begging) without raising the Price of Cattle, and of Corn, although they should live upon Chaff. Hence our encrease of Buildings in this City, because Workmen have nothing to do but employ one another, and one half of them are infallibly undone. Hence the daily encrease of *Bankers*, who may be a necessary Evil in a Trading-Country, but so ruinous in Ours, who for their private Advantage have sent away all our Silver, and one third of our Gold, so that within three Years past, the

running

running Caſh of the Nation, which was about Five hundred thouſand Pounds, is now leſs than two, and muſt daily diminiſh unleſs we have Liberty to Coin, as well as that important Kingdom the Iſle of *Man*, and the meaneſt Prince in the *German Empire*, as I before obſerved.

I have ſometimes thought, that this Paradox of the Kingdom growing Rich, is chiefly owing to thoſe worthy Gentlemen the BANKERS, who, except ſome Cuſtom-houſe Officers, Birds of Paſſage, oppreſſive thrifty 'Squires, and a few others that ſhall be Nameleſs, are the only thriving People among us: And I have often wiſhed that a Law were enacted to hang up half a Dozen *Bankers* every year, and thereby interpoſe at leaſt ſome ſhort Delay, to the further Ruin of *Ireland*.

Ye are idle, ye are idle, anſwered *Pharoah* to the *Iſraelites*, when they complained to his MAJESTY, that they were forced to make Bricks without Straw.

England enjoys every one of theſe Advantages for enriching a Nation, which I have above enumerated, and into the Bargain, a good Million returned to them every Year without Labour or Hazard, or one Farthing value received on our ſide. But how long we ſhall be able to continue the payment, I

am

am not under the leaſt Concern. One thing I know, that *when the Hen is ſtarved to Death, there will be no more Golden Eggs.*

I think it a little unhoſpitable, and others may call it a ſubtil piece of Malice, that, becauſe there may be a Dozen Families in this Town, able to entertain their *Engliſh* Friends in a generous manner at their Tables, their Gueſts upon their Return to *England*, ſhall report that we wallow in Riches and Luxury.

Yet I confeſs I have known an Hoſpital, where all the Houſehold-Officers grew Rich, while the Poor for whoſe ſake it was built, were almoſt ſtarving for want of Food and Raiment.

To Conclude. If *Ireland* be a rich and flouriſhing Kindgom, it's Wealth and Proſperity muſt be owing to certain Cauſes, that are yet concealed from the whole Race of Mankind, and the Effects are equally Inviſible. We need not wonder at Strangers when they deliver ſuch Paradoxes, but a Native and Inhabitant of this Kingdom, who gives the ſame Verdict, muſt be either ignorant to Stupidity, or a Man-pleaſer at the Expence of all Honour, Conſcience and Truth.

FINIS

Rutty (1770)
A Chronological History of the Weather and Seasons

John Rutty, *A Chronological History of the Weather and Seasons, and of the Prevailing Diseases in Dublin. With their Various Periods, Successions, and Revolutions, during the Space of Forty Years. With a Comparative View of the Difference of the Irish Climate and Diseases, and those of England and other Countries* (London: Robinson and Roberts, 1770).

John Rutty (1698–1775) was born into a Quaker family in Wiltshire and remained a member of the Society of Friends throughout his life. He studied medicine at the University of Leiden, graduating MD in 1723 and in the following year he settled in Dublin. John Rutty was admitted as a Licentiate Fellow of the King and Queen's College of Physicians in 1729 and took an active part in the intellectual life of the city. He was a member of the Physico-Historical Society (1744–52) established to survey the 'antient and present state' of Irish counties and in 1755 became a founder member of the Medio-Philosophical Society.[1] An eventual outcome as part of the former activity was his *Essay towards a Natural History of the County of Dublin* published in 1772.[2] He was also a member of the short-lived Botanical Society of Ireland.

Rutty had three life-long interests. The first was the Society of Friends and in 1751 he published a revised edition of Thomas Wright's history of the Society.[3] His second was natural history. This included investigations into the chemical composition and medicinal properties of mineral waters that resulted in *A Methodi-*

1. Eoin Magennis, '"A Land of Milk and Honey": the Physio-Historical Society, Improvement and the Surveys of Mid-Eighteenth Century Ireland', *Proceedings of the Royal Irish Academy*, 102C:6 (2002), pp. 204, 206.

2. John Rutty, *An Essay towards a Natural History of the County of Dublin, Accomodated to the Noble Designs of the Dublin Society* ... (Dublin: W. Sleater, 1772).

3. Thomas Wright, *History of the Rise and Progress of the People called Quakers in Ireland, from 1653 to 1700 ... first compiled by T. W. ... Now revised and enlarged. To which is added a continuation ... to ... 1751. With an Introduction ... and a Treatise of the Christian Discipline exercised among the said People, by J. Rutty* (Dublin: I. Jackson, 1751).

cal Synopsis of Mineral Waters (1757) and several papers in the *Transactions of the Royal Society*.[1] It also embraced his interest in the weather and seasons, which spilled over into his third concern: the nature of epidemic diseases. The two came together in his *Chronological History of the Weather and Seasons*.

The *Chronological History* has a simple thesis: that there is a connection between weather and disease. Rutty argued that the nature and severity of epidemics varied according to the weather, at least in the countryside; in the cities the smoke of the fires interfered with the relationship, on the whole for the better. Different diseases prevailed in different climates; and different seasons within the same climate produced different diseases. The weather affected the propagation of diseases, although it could not explain their causes. The bulk of the diseases confronting Rutty in Ireland were fevers of various kinds, 'anginas' (mostly sore throats but also chest pains), eye infections, diarrhoea and dysentery, and catarrh. There were sporadic outbreaks of smallpox

The recording of weather in a systematic manner had developed during the seventeenth and eighteenth centuries as men tried to understand the natural world. The discipline of making precise observations fitted in well with Rutty's religious practices that led him to keep a daily spiritual diary that was published after his death.[2] The interest by physicians in the connection between climate and disease goes back to Hippocrates, although Rutty's immediate inspiration was Thomas Sydenham who published his *Observationes Medicae* in 1676.[3] His debt to Sydenham was acknowledged by Rutty's description of him as 'the divine old man'.[4]

The chief interest of the *Chronological History* for Irish historians is its discussion of diseases during the famine of 1740–1. At the end of December 1739 Ireland was gripped by a biting frost that ushered in twenty-one months of the most sustained cold ever expe-

1. John Rutty, *A Methodical Synopsis of Mineral Waters, Comprehending the Most Celebrated Medicinal Waters, both cold and hot ... and Abstracts of the Principal Authors who have treated of Mineral Waters, etc.* (London: William Johnston, 1757).

2. Jan Golinski, 'Putting the Weather in Order: Narrative and Discipline in Eighteenth-Century Weather Diaries'. Paper given at the William Andrews Clark Memorial Library, UCLA, Los Angeles, May 1998 (available online). Brian Hill, 'A Spiritual Diarist: John Rutty, M.D. 1698–1775', *The Practitioner*, 187 (1961), pp. 219–23.

3. C.S. Breathnach, 'Doctor John Rutty [1698–1777]: Medicine and Meteorology', *Journal of the Irish Colleges of Physicians and Surgeons*, 29:2 (2000), pp. 106–8.

4. John Rutty, *A Chronological History of the Weather and Seasons, and of the Prevailing Diseases in Dublin. With their Various Periods, Successions, and Revolutions, during the Space of Forty Years. With a Comparative View of the Difference of the Irish Climate and Diseases, and those of England and other Countries* (London: Robinson and Roberts, 1770), p. 236.

rienced in north-western Europe. The potato and grain harvests were ruined, unemployment was rife, and between 310,000 and 480,000 people out of a population of 2.4 million may have perished from starvation and disease.[1] Rutty catalogued the various fevers prevalent at the time and provided the first clear description of relapsing fever, a louse-transmitted infection that ravaged the starving population. In the words of one authority, 'Rutty's account is a textbook description of the clinical course of relapsing fever as it has occurred in the British Isles'.[2]

1. David Dickson, *Arctic Ireland. The Extraordinary Story of the Great Frost and Forgotten Famine of 1740–41* (Belfast: White Row Press, 1997).

2. John D. Post, *Food Shortage, Climatic Variability, and Epidemic Disease in Preindustrial Europe. The Mortality Peak in the early 1740s* (Ithaka: Cornell University Press, 1985), p. 244.

A

CHRONOLOGICAL HISTORY

OF THE

WEATHER AND SEASONS,

And of the Prevailing

DISEASES IN DUBLIN.

WITH

Their various PERIODS, SUCCESSIONS, and REVOLUTIONS, during the SPACE of Forty YEARS.

WITH

A comparative VIEW of the DIFFERENCE of the IRISH CLIMATE and DISEASES, and thoſe of ENGLAND and other COUNTRIES.

By JOHN RUTTY, M.D.

LONDON:

Printed for ROBINSON and ROBERTS, N°. 25, in PATER-NOSTER-ROW.

MDCCLXX.

PREFACE.

THAT faithful hiſtories of the ſtate of the air and weather peculiar to any country may be of real uſe, as a branch of natural hiſtory, and be a means of confirming or of correcting divers eſtabliſhed opinions relative hereto, will not be denied; nor that a daily record of the various changes of the air, weather, and winds, is abſolutely neceſſary for this purpoſe.

From ſuch a regiſtry, it will appear that even in this changeable climate, cer-

certain ſtated revolutions (although often interrupted) of the weather and winds may be traced through the ſeveral ſeaſons of the year; and ſuch revolutions as are highly worthy the attention of valetudinarians as well as phyſicians, and of the laſt more eſpecially, by accounts of the concomitant diſeaſes annexed, whereby ſomething of a like periodical revolution in them alſo may be diſcovered ſo far that the return of ſome of them at certain ſeaſons is almoſt as certain as that of ſwallows in ſummer; and it may be ſhewn how far certain diſeaſes, and their propagation, duration, increaſe, and the degrees of their malignity, have a connexion with the ſtate of the air and weather attending, which is one principal ſcope of the preſent Work. But it ſhall ſuffice in this place to obſerve, with reſpect to the

the influence of the ſeaſons in general, that in ſpring the vegetables put forth their buds, the birds renew their ſongs, the ſleeping animals and inſects come forth, and moſt of the quadrupeds, and even the inhabitants of the deep, are not inſenſible of its influence *; as neither is the human body, their being ſeveral evidences of a greater ſwell in the tide of the circulating fluid of that ſeaſon, though the winds from the north and eaſt, uſually attending it, frequently prove very noxious not only to vegetables, but to men, particularly valetudinarians, as in the following pages will abundantly appear; and that fevers are more frequent with us in winter than in ſummer, which may be partly attributed to the comparative

* See Thompſon on the Seaſons.

warmth

warmth of the former ſeaſon, and the coolneſs of the latter, peculiar to us.

This method of treating of diſeaſes was purſued by the father of phyſic, and has lately been revived by ſeveral Engliſh writers, particularly Wintringham, Huxham, and the indefatigable Dr. Short. The obſervations of theſe authors, I have frequently, in the courſe of this Work, compared with my own, and confirmed them; and I truſt that the longer ſeries of time to which mine were protracted may add more weight to the evidence of the truth of the conſequences drawn from ſuch compariſon.

The compiler of the following Obſervations thinks proper to acknow-

ledge

ledge that the principal ſubjects of them were not what an eminent brother calls *ſplendidæ perſonæ*, but plebeians, and *mediæ ſortis homines*: a circumſtance however, which, in his apprehenſion, ought rather to recommend than diſparage the work; inaſmuch as theſe laſt named perſons are more expoſed to the injuries of the air and weather than the other, who, by means of their warm cloathing, good fires, and the moderate uſe of wine, are leſs ſuſceptible thereof: to which add that in them alſo the genuine proceſs of nature, in the conduct and cure of diſeaſes, is commonly not ſo much diſguiſed by art as where leſs is committed to nature.

The following account has been drawn up from diaries conſtantly kept both

both of the weather and diſeaſes; but as the prolixity and tedioufneſs of diaries, on the one hand, would deter moſt men from reading them, and, on the other, the vagueneſs and obſcurity of even quarterly or yearly accounts, are ſuch as would not give proper ſatisfaction to an inquiſitive mind, I have reduced the diaries of the weather to the form of monthly regiſtries; and greatly contracted the accounts of the diſeaſes.

In the following Hiſtory of the Diſeaſes particular regard is had to the duration of the ſeveral fevers, the number of days in which they terminated being ſpecified with as much preciſion as practicable. It is true, the firſt commencement of a fever is often very hard to be determined: however, the reckoning was uſually made

made from the firſt ſhivering to the time when the pulſe fell to the healthful ſtandard of its velocity, or rather below it. This has been done with a view to the ancient doctrine of critical days; and to ſhew, that even in this changeable climate, ſome attention hereunto may be of uſe to the phyſician, both in his prognoſtications and his conduct in the cure of fevers, it being a ſettled point that any evacuation by ſtool, ſweat, hemorrhage, or any remarkable change of the urine, are of more efficacy when they occur on the critical days than on the intermediate days.

Now the ſummary reſult of the obſervations in the following Work in reſpect to this matter, is, that amidſt all the obſcurities and uncertainties attending the ſeventh, fourteenth, twen-

twentieth, and twenty-firſt days, were nearly either the days of the moſt perfect criſis, or the days on which the greateſt number of fevers terminated either in the recovery or death of the patient. It is true, many of our fevers did alſo terminate in five or ſix days: but the criſis in this caſe was commonly imperfect, the patients being ſubject to relapſes.

And it is allowed by a certain eminent profeſſor, that, although indeed every day may prove a critical one, yet that the ſeventh, fourteenth, and twentieth are the principal of the critical days: and to this agrees an aphoriſm left us by an author in a very remote country, Paulus Ægineta, viz. *Dies judicatorii optimi ſunt ſeptimus & decimus quartus*; and a later one of Fernelius, viz.

Con-

Continuam febrem ſecunda, aut (quod tardiſſimum eſt) tertia hebdomada decretori, ſolvit; and in Hippocrates's Epidemics, the greateſt number finiſhed their courſe in ſeven, the next in fourteen days, the next in twenty-one days nearly, though ſome few of his, with their relapſes, continued above two months, as with us: but this is very rare, and, according to Fernelius, muſt be owing to unſound viſcera: from all which it appears that the veneration paid by antiquity to the number ſeven was not altogether without foundation.

And it is hoped that the following conſiderations may recommend the Work to younger phyſicians, viz. as, during the term of theſe obſervations, we have been four times viſited in Dublin with an epidemic contagion of foreign original, the catarrhal fever, which

which was a ſignal inſtance of the influence of the air and weather on diſeaſes, according to the ſeveral ſeaſons in which it appeared; and although not attended with any extraordinary malignity, yet once, in a ſeaſon favouring its progreſs, raiſed our bills of mortality to three times their uſual number: it therefore ſeemed to be of real uſe that ſome record ſhould be preſerved of it, and its method of cure, as matter of inſtruction on any like future emergency.

And moreover, as another diſeaſe, little leſs than peſtilential, attacked our children, eſpecially in the country in the year 1743, five years before Dr. Fothergill publiſhed his accurate account of a diſeaſe near akin to it in the neighbourhood of London,

don, but much milder, though nothing ever tranſpired from hence in a publick manner concerning it, ſome account of it, and ſome practical hints are here given, which it is hoped will not be unacceptable nor uſeleſs; and if to this I ſhould add the direful conſequences of the great froſt 1739, 1740, more pernicious than ſome peſtilences, it is to be hoped that no further apology need be made for the preſent publication.

N. B. I have begun my year with March, as being, notwithſtanding our alteration of ſtyle, ſtill the firſt month of the ſpring-quarter, and January and February the two laſt of the winter-quarter, and agreeing neareſt in temperature to December, which I reckon ſtill the firſt month of the winter-

winter-quarter; and ſo February with me terminates every year, and January and February, inſtead of being the two firſt months of any given year, are the two laſt of the ſame year with me.

INTRODUCTION.

PART I.

Shewing the Influence of the Air and Weather on Diſeaſes.

IN order for the conviction of thoſe who are crying down any attempts to trace a connection between the ſtate of the air and weather, and the prevailing epidemics, eſpecially in this changeable climate, I ſhall endeavour to ſhew in the following pages, and in the courſe of this Work, that both the endemial and epidemic diſeaſes of different countries are very different in their type, duration, and degree of malignity, according to the

the different ſtate of the air and weather in thoſe ſeveral countries, and according to the different ſeaſons in the ſame country.

I. It is to the difference of the air in cities and in country places that epidemic fevers commonly make a far greater havock in the laſt, where a depraved conſtitution of the air produces the moſt pernicious effects: whereas in cities the air is altered, and in ſome ſort corrected, by the fires and other effluvia.

II. Different diſeaſes prevail in different climates, ſuitable to the different temperature of the air in thoſe ſeveral climates *. Thus agues are obſerved to be the great endemic of all moiſt countries: and whereas Dr. Mead makes this general and important obſervation,

* Linnæus remarks, that neither the deſtructive plagues among men, which are very frequent in hotter countries, nor even poiſonous plants or animals, are ſo frequent in the regions of the north as in thoſe of the ſouth.

that

that no kind of putrefaction bred here in these European countries is ever heightened to the degree capable of producing the plague; on the contrary, in Asia and other hotter countries, and where the humors are more disposed to putrefaction, and the fibres more crisp and contracted, ardent, pestilential, and contagious fevers are much more frequent, and even endemial; and their fevers finish their course with much more rapidity than in these islands, placed in a cold and moist air, and where, as it is observable in Huxham's History of the prevailing Diseases at Plymouth, for ten years, that defluxions, coughs, tumors of the jaws, opthalmies, and anginas, fill up near three-fourths of the catalogue, which is also the case here; so that these may be said to be our endemial diseases common to both countries, as islands in a like cold and moist situation, and subject unto the like vicissitudes of weather.

And

And if the moiſture of the air proper to us ſhould predominate long, and eſpecially if warmth ſhould conſpire with it, catarrhal, intermittent, ſlow, nervous, and petechial fevers have been obſerved to prevail. This was notoriouſly the caſe at Dublin and Cork, on a compariſon of Dr. Rogers's account of the epidemic, low, putrid fever, which was common to both cities at the ſame time; and that author obſerves, that for a ſeries of near twenty years preceding the year 1734, no new epidemic fever ſhewed itſelf among them at Cork, but of the ſame kind which hath been very frequent here ſince that time, eſpecially in ſuch ſeaſons as are before mentioned; from which and other ſimilar obſervations, joined to the following deſcription of the malignant fever moſt common in Ireland, left us in Boate's Natural Hiſtory, publiſhed above a hundred years ago, the fever of the low putrid kind appears to be endemial to us, viz.

"It

" It is common to the natives and to thofe who come thither from other countries. It is commonly attended with a great pain of the head and in all the bones, great weaknefs, reftleffnefs, ravings, but no very great nor conftant heat, and it is hard to be cured; and the cure is not to be effected by purging, which cannot be ufed at any time without great danger, and hardly by bleeding, which is feldom ufed with fuccefs, except at the very beginning; but by ftrengthening medicines and good cordials, and in fome years an extraordinary and peftilent malignity cometh to it, with fo great violence that, notwithftanding all good helps, fome are thereby carried to their graves."

It is well known that thefe fevers frequently run out to the length of three weeks or fometimes a month: on the contrary, how much more violent and how much more rapid in their courfe their fevers in the hot countries are, will appear from the following detail.

1. In

1. In the Eaſt Indies Bontius deſcribes their continual fevers thus: *Plerumque; cum tanto furore hic mortales invadunt, ut tanquam attonitos, de ratione mentis ſtatim dejiciant, & ſæpe intra pauciſſimos dies, imo aliquando horas, cum phrenitide ac continuo delirio ægros e vita rapiant: adſunt perpetuæ vigiliæ, vomitus varii coloris, præcipue viridis ac æruginoſæ bilis. Externa rigent: calor internus cum ingenti ſiti vitales ac naturales facultates depaſcitur.*

2. In Egypt, Proſper Alpinus obſerves, that during the ſeaſon of their periodical hot winds, attended alſo with a changeable ſtate of the weather, from September till June, the plague rages every year; as alſo peſtilential fevers and phrenzies, which kill in a few hours; whereas Galen never obſerved phreneticks to die before the third day, and at the ſame time alſo rages a peſtilential ſmall pox among children: but this ſeaſon is ſucceeded by the cold north winds in June, and an uniform ſtate of weather; and

and then the plague and most other diseases vanish.

3. In Minorca (a hot country, where Farenheit's thermometer rises to eighty-two and eighty-seven) acute fevers are more frequent than in England, and withal much more violent, but of shorter duration: they oftener terminate completely by a manifest crisis, and in all respects agree much more exactly with what the antients have said concerning such evacuations and the periods in which they happen *.

4. The ardent bilious fever in Barbadoes (being common to Siam, situated in the same latitude as Dr. Hilary observes †) usually terminates about the

* Cleghorn's Observations on the Diseases of Minorca.

† Dr. Hilary observes that this fever is found there in all seasons. He also describes the slow nervous fever, common to us and them, running out to the nineteenth, twentieth, and twenty-first days, terminating sometimes with and sometimes without a manifest crisis, but which is rare there; insomuch that from 1754 to 1758, it entirely disappeared.

fourth

fourth day from the attack, the regular crisis generally discovering itself by a suffusion of the bile over the surface of the body the third day *.

5. In Carthagena in America, situated in 10°. 25′. N. latitude, where their heats are excessive, without receiving any sensible mitigation from the nights, the distempers that attack the Europeans are very dangerous, and their continuance is very short, viz. they last but three or four days, in which time the sick either die or are out of danger †.

But more particularly, to shew how much the regularity of the diseases prevailing in different countries depends on the regularity of their respective seasons and weather, and *vice versa*.

1. In Greece, and in Asia in general, where their seasons are for the most part uniform, and their winds periodical, the

* Towne on the Diseases of the West Indies.

† Philos. Transactions. N° 492.

dif-

difference of their ſeaſons and their effects were more eaſily obſerved *.

Hence Hippocrates, l. 3. prog. 8. *Cum anni tempus propriam habet temperaturam morbi fiunt conſtantes & optimi judicii.*

And I apprehend that an impartial attention to the following hiſtories of the ſeaſons and their concomitant diſeaſes will ſhew, that the obſervations of Hippocrates with regard to the ſeaſons and diſeaſes, do alſo, allowance being made for the difference of the climate, in a great meaſure, hold good here. His ſummary account of this matter is,

Quod hyems corpus pituitâ repleat, inde cognoſcere datur, quod homines pituitoſiſſima & ſpuunt & emungunt hyeme, & tumores laxi & albiſſimi fiunt, maxime hoc tempore, itemque; reliqui morbi pituitoſi.

Vere Sanguis augeſcit.

* Mead Monita & Præc. Medica.

Homi-

Homines vere & æstate maxime dysenteriis corripiuntur, & sanguis ex naribus ipsis fluit. At vero æstate sanguis adhuc viget & bilis in corpore elevatur, & usque in autumnum porrigitur. In autumno autem sanguis modicus fit: bilis autem per æstatem ac autumnum possidet; id quod inde cognoscere potes, quod homines, sua sponte hoc tempore bilem evomunt, & in medicamentorum purgationibus biliosiora purgentur: manifestum fit & febribus & hominum caloribus.

Atra bilis autumno & plurima & fortissima est. Lib. de Natura Hominis.

And again, *Morbi omnes quidem in omnibus temporibus fiunt; quidam tamen magis in quibusdam ipsorum & fiunt & exacerbantur. Vere etenim insaniæ & atræ biles & comitiales, & sanguinis fluxiones, & anginæ, & gravedines, & raucedines, & tusses, & lepræ & impetigines, & vitiligines, & pustulæ ulcerosæ plurimæ, & tubercula & morbus articularis.*

Aestate

Aeſtate vero & quidam ex his, & febres continuæ, & ardentes, & tertianæ plurime & quartane & vomitus, & alvi profluvia, & lippitudines & aurium dolores & oris exulcerationes, & pudendorem putredines & papulæ ſudoroſæ. Autumno autem & ex æſtivis multi, & febres quartanæ & erroneæ, & ſplenes; & hydropes, & tabes, & urinæ ſtillicidia; & inteſtinorum lævitates & dyſenteriæ, & coxendices, & anginæ & anhelationes, & volvuli & comitiales, & inſaniæ & atræ biles.

Hyeme vero pleuritides, peripneumoniæ & gravedines, raucedines, tuſſes, dolores pectorum, laterum ac lumborum, capitis dolores, vertigines, ſyderationes.

2. At Charles-town, in South Carolina, their epidemic diſeaſes return as regularly at their ſtated ſeaſons as a good clock ſtrikes twelve when the ſun is in the meridian, viz. in July, Auguſt, and September, when great heat and moiſture prevail *.

* Phil. Tranſ. Nº 470.

3. In

3. In the Eaſt-Indies, when there are perpetual rains with great heat, viz. from November till May, it is ſickly; and contra, from May to October, as it is dry, ſerene, and cooler, it is alſo healthier *. And ſo,

4. In Minorca remittent and intermittent fevers return with the utmoſt regularity every July, and continue till October or November, and do not return till next July, agreeable to the conſtancy of their weather, which is for the moſt part very hot and dry all ſummer; but the diſeaſes of the winter and ſpring, agreeable to the various diſpoſitions of thoſe ſeaſons, are neither ſo uniform nor certain †. What then are we to expect here but variety of diſeaſes, and particularly of fevers, and irregularity and uncertainty in their types and periods, agreeable to the changeable ſtate of the ſeaſons and weather proper to our climate?

* Bond. Med. Indor.

† Cleghorn loc. cit.

which

which accordingly is the caſe. Nevertheleſs,

III. Different ſeaſons of the year, even in the ſame climate, are attended with different diſeaſes, and have notable effects in promoting or checking their propagation.

There ſeems to be in the ſpring ſome greater degree of ebullition in the blood; whence puſtules and ſome other diſorders latent in winter appear, and ſcrophulous ſores are obſerved to break out afreſh, or to appear in greater numbers; and pleuriſies and other inflammatory diſorders commonly attend the cold northerly winds frequent in that ſeaſon, when alſo tertian agues are frequent, according to the poet,

> Each changing ſeaſon doth its poiſon bring,
> Rheums chill the winter, agues blaſt the ſpring.
>
> PRIOR.

Which though it generally holds here alſo, yet we find not unfrequently coughs and defluxions to attend the ſummer on changeable wind and weather; and that theſe diſorders

orders are the confequence of a change, not only from heat to cold, but of cold to heat.

There feems alfo to be in fome degree fomething periodical in the return of the *colera morbus*, diarrhœas, and fometimes dyfenteries at the end of fummer and in autumn, but uncertainly, agreeable to the variablenefs of the temperature of the air and weather here; and our fummers (frequently winter-like) are fo far from being diftinguifhed by the greater prevalence of fevers, that the winter in general (here frequently warm, and confiderably more fo than in England) has the greater number, although the fummer fometimes has more than the fpring and fall, as is elfewhere obferved.

This may be owing to the coolnefs and temperatenefs of our fummers, more remarkable indeed than in Great Britain.

Dr. Pringle, in his Obfervations on the Difeafes of the Army, remarks fomething very like this with refpect to the fummers

mers of Great-Britain, which, I think, well worth tranſcribing here, as a confirmation and further illuſtration of this reaſoning.

"In the Netherlands, where the weather in ſummer is hotter, and in winter colder than in England, the epidemic diſeaſes may be dated from ſome time in July, or the beginning of Auguſt, under the canicular heats *, their ſenſible decline about the fall of the leaf, and end when the froſts begin; and their ſummer and autumnal diſeaſes are intermitting and remitting fevers, diarrhœas, and dyſenteries; but the diſeaſes of winter are inflammatory, as colds in various ſhapes, coughs, ſtitches, rheumatic pains, pleuriſies, inflammations of the lungs, &c. which continue throughout the ſpring,

* The bile and other animal humours are exalted by this means. So the bite of the tarantula, and of the ſcorpion, is not venomous in winter, but in ſummer only; and Celſus remarks ſerpents to be more venomous in hot countries.

and

and till paſt the ſummer-ſolſtice; though towards the ſummer-ſolſtice, as the weather grows warmer, the colds are not attended with coughs, ſtitches, and diſorders of the breaſt, but rather a continued fever."

Then, in making the compariſon between Great-Britain and the Netherlands, he obſerves, that, remitting and intermitting fevers, and the dyſentery, which are periodical, and rage with much worſe ſymptoms, from the more intenſe heat and moiſture in the Netherlands, are more gentle, and ſeldom epidemic in Great-Britain, (except in extraordinary cloſe and hot ſeaſons) which are ſeldom of long continuance there, and in the fenny tracts, by reaſon of the comparative dryneſs of the ſoil, its freedom from marſhes, the conſtant perflation, and the moderate and interrupted heat of our ſummers; and that our blood is liable but to a ſmall degree of putrid acrimony to what theirs is in the hotter countries: and what Sanctorius

torius ſays of the winters in Italy is more or leſs applicable to all the ſeaſons in Great-Britain, viz. *Adiapneuſtia quæ æſtate febrem malignam, hyeme vix minimam alterationem efficere poteſt, corpora enim acriore perſpirabili æſtate referta ſunt quam hyeme.*

Now if all this be true of England, it will hold ſtill more in Ireland, where our ſummers are remarkably more cool and temperate.

IV. That the weather has a powerful immediate influence, if not in the generation, at leaſt in the propagation, increaſe, and abatement of diſeaſes, further appears alſo from hence.

There is ſcarce any phyſician converſant in practice here but muſt have obſerved a remarkable greater degree of healthineſs when in a ſummer ſeaſon the weather ſets in for fair and ſerene for a conſiderable time; as likewiſe that any great, notable, and ſudden changes of weather, (as particularly a ſudden onſet of winter) are generally followed by a far

greater

greater frequency of colds and inflammatory diſorders: but more particularly

The greater or leſs fatality of the epidemic catarrhal fever, with which we have been four times viſited within the compaſs of theſe obſervations, was remarkably influenced by the ſeveral reſpective ſeaſons in which it invaded us; for when it came in October 1737, the weekly bill of mortality at its greateſt height roſe to a hundred forty-four; when it came in May 1743, it roſe only to ſixty-ſeven; when in February and March 1732-3, to ninety-eight, viz. according to the different warmth of the ſeveral ſeaſons encouraging or diſcouraging the diſcharge by the ſkin, which was the natural criſis.

Again, that in a ſerene and dry ſtate of the air, whether very hot or very cold, long continued inflammatory fevers prevail; and that in moiſt and warm conſtitutions of the air, long, intermitting, ſlow, putrid, and malignant fevers, prevail,

prevail, is agreed by all obſervers; which was notoriouſly the caſe here alſo in the rainy years of 1734, 1735, when our ſummers were like winters, and our winters wanted their uſual cold and froſt. Such was the ſtate of the weather here, and in England at that time; and in both places the ſame kind of diſeaſes greatly prevailed, viz. the intermittent, remittent, and ſlow nervous fever, which diſorders were remarkably baniſhed by the great froſt of 1739, 1740, and the ſucceeding dry ſeaſon 1740, 1741; in the hiſtory of which, in its proper place, I have, ſhewn that this and the moſt celebrated of the other great froſts were attended with ſimilar diſeaſes; and an ague was ſcarcely to be ſeen, until the return of the rainy and moiſt ſeaſons, 1744, 1745, with which the intermittents returned, and became the prevailing diſeaſe.

But in our reaſonings on the operation of the weather in promoting epidemic diſ-

diſeaſes, we are to conſider its paſt as well as preſent ſtate. Thus catarrhs, coughs, hoarſeneſſes, head-achs, and other diſorders depending on the lymph, are not always the immediate effect of a preſent moiſt temperature of the air, nor do ſometimes happen until a cold and dry temperature ſucceeds, which ſhutting up the pores, retains and coagulates the redundant moiſture collected in the preceding ſeaſon; and ſo dyſenteries have attended a cold and moiſt, ſucceeded by a hot intemperature of the air, the firſt ſtopping perſpiration and accumulating a collection of ſerous humours, and the laſt ſeting them in action, and ſometimes *vice verſa*: on which account the worſt effects of the great froſt in 1739, 1740, did not appear until the thaw.

Upon the whole, it abundantly appears, that the different ſtate of the air is one principal fomes of the variety of epidemic diſeaſes, and yet not the ſole, but

other

other non-naturals, and particularly the diet is to be admitted as a confiderable co-operating caufe, efpecially in the dearth and badnefs of provifions; as in the years 1728, 1729, in the North, and 1741 throughout the kingdom.

PART

PART II.

Of the Air and Weather of Ireland in General, and their Influence on the Health and Diſeaſes of the Inhabitants, and ſome Things peculiar to it.

THE air of Ireland, in general, hath not unjuſtly obtained the reputation of being peculiarly wholeſome and healthful, not only becauſe no poſitive inſtance hath been produced of any venomous creature being found in it, but there ſeems to be ſomething in it that reſiſts the propagation of diſeaſes, if not alſo of poiſonous animals, more than in the air of ſome neighbouring countries: however, Boate, in his Natural Hiſtory of Ireland, obſerves, that the plague which did ſo often and cruelly infeſt England, was wonderfully rare in Ireland, and ſcarce ſeen once in an age. Per-

Perhaps our acute diſeaſes are generally leſs violent and leſs inflammatory than for the moſt part in England: however, I have been not only aſſured that the epidemic diſorder called the Dunkirk fever, was milder and leſs mortal here than in England; but can take upon me to affirm, that, on comparing the deſcriptions of two epidemic diſorders which were common to both countries, and raged at the ſame time in both, the ſymptoms were much milder, and the diſeaſes leſs mortal here than in England. The dyſentery, which in hot countries makes frequent returns, and often dreadful ravages, ſeldom viſits us in an epidemic way. The dry belly-ach, the tetanus, and opiſthotonos, frequent alſo and often mortal, and the elephantiaſis and lepra arabum, ſo frequent in the hot climates, are ſcarce known among us; and even the *rabies canina* is alſo much leſs frequent than in England; and the healthineſs of our climate in general appears from the rarity of of any notable depopulating epidemics among us, ſo great that, during a reſidence of above forty years in the practice of phyſic in Dublin, I remember but three or four remarkable inſtances of ſuch.

Our weather indeed is extremely variable, and its changes often ſudden; and yet the changes, and their conſequent effects, are far leſs conſiderable than what Piſo notes of the Weſt-Indies, and Bontius of the Eaſt, and Proſper Alpinus of Egypt, with reſpect to the extreme coldneſs of their evenings ſucceeding the intenſe heat of their days, to the great prejudice of the health of men.

And whereas in Dublin the variation of Fahrenheit's thermometer in twenty-four hours ſcarce exceeds five or ſix degrees, in South-Carolina there have been obſerved thirty degrees difference in twenty-four hours in that inſtrument, the variation of which there alſo is eighty-three degrees; but here, during the courſe of

one

one year, it did not exceed thirty-ſix degrees (in another about forty-eight, varying from twenty-ſeven to ſeventy-five.)

Here it is to be obſerved that the long duration of the twilight in our oblique ſphere contributes much to make the tranſition from the heat of the day to the damp of the evening far leſs ſudden than in other ſituations, v. g. in Barbadoes, where the right aſcent and deſcent of the ſun makes that tranſition far more quick than in Europe.

At the ſame time our weather is generally more free from great exceſſes of heat and cold than theirs in England, from our ſituation farther out in the ocean: hence the ſnow lies but a little while here, and it hails but ſeldom, and in thin and ſhort ſhowers, and the hail-ſtones are ſo very ſmall *, that the authentic accounts we have from England of ſome of their hail-ſtones being ſix inches, and ſome nine

* Boate's Nat. Hiſt. of Ireland.

inches

inches in circumference, and ſome that lately fell at Williamſburg in Virginia as big as hens eggs, and others as big as gooſe eggs, and proving fatal to partridges, hares, cattle, and people *, would ſeem almoſt incredible to us, were not theſe accounts further confirmed by divine authority in the ſacred writings; † where we read that God deſtroyed the enemies of Iſrael with hail-ſtones, which killed more than the children of Iſrael ſlew with the ſword; and whilſt I am on the praiſes of this iſland, it were injuſtice to be ſilent as to our comparative exemption, not only from the dreadful hurricanes that frequently infeſt our colonies, but even from the violent ſtorms which we frequently hear of from England, tearing up trees by the roots, &c. which are but rarely felt here to that degree.

The comparative heat of the ſeveral ſeaſons in London and Dublin is thus

* Short's Chron. Hiſt. † Joſhua X.

eſtimated

eſtimated by that curious obſerver Dr. Bryan Robinſon *.

	In London.	In Dublin
Winter	1.00	1.45
Spring	3.00	2.14
Summer	5.00	4.68
Autumn	3.00	3.80
	12.00	12.07

This greater warmth of our air than is common to ſo northern a ſituation is probably the cauſe why the perſpiration of the human body is ſo great here, viz. which being eſtimated at a medium for the whole year in Dublin 1721 and 1744, on a compariſon made in the ſeveral places under-mentioned, was as follows:

* Obſervations on the Virtues and Operations of Medicines.

In

In Dublin,	1721	1.141
	1744	0.980
In Cork		1.472
In England		0.817
In South Carolina		0.927
In Italy		1.480

From whence it ſhould appear that the perſpiration in Ireland is greater than in England; and in South Carolina, and in Corke, almoſt equal to what it is in Italy.

But though our air be temperate as to heat and cold, the country has not unjuſtly acquired the appellation of *matula Jovis*, from its redundant moiſture, eaſily accounted for from our ſituation farther out in the ocean, and our nearer approach to the vapours brought to us on the wings of our predominant W. and S. W. winds, and eſpecially more peculiarly from ſome point of the ſouth, more than about London, as appears from Diaries of the weather kept in both places.

The

The ſignal moiſture of our air further appears from our frequent wet ſummers, more like winter, from our fogs in winter, frequently ſo loaded with vapours, as not only to increaſe the weight of the hygrometer, but to raiſe the mercury in the barometer; and as a further proof of the great moiſture of our air, the firſt named inſtrument varied in its weight in ſeveral years from two hundred forty-one to four hundred and thirty-three, viz. a hundred and ninety-two grains.

Our linen and our paper imbibe this moiſture, books grow mouldy, our woollen alſo in rooms without a fire imbibe it, even in ſummer time; ſo do ſalt, ſugar, hops, meal; and our corn requires to be kiln-dried, (a practice in a manner unknown in ſome parts of England) and Boyle Godfrey, the chymiſt, affirmed, that the fixed ſalts imbibe much more moiſture here than in London; and a traveller of veracity aſſures me, that the icicles dangling on our hair in travelling here

here in frosty weather, are not observed on the continent of America, as a proof of the abundance of watery vapours suspended in our air: from all which it is evident, that we live in a constant *balneum vaporis*, which undoubtedly is also imbibed by the absorbent vessels on the surface of our bodies.

This moisture and temperate quality of our air is, however, in some respects, a great advantage to us, whilst it secures us both from the pernicious effects of excessive heat and drought, productive in warmer climates of much more acute and more violently inflammatory disorders than are found here; but likewise from the ill effects of excessive cold and dryness, not less remarkable for the production of inflammatory diseases than heat and dryness, as appears by repeated observations.

The watery vapours with which our air abounds serve, in some measure, to qualify the crisping drying quality of our E. N. and N. E. winds, and at the same time yield a constant fomentation to our fibres, and

and being imbibed at the cutaneous pores• dilute our blood: to which agrees well an obſervation of the above cited late Dr. Bryan Robinſon *, viz. " In the mortal inflammatory fever deſcribed by Tabor, the ſpecific gravity of the ſerum was nearly ten thouſand four hundred and eight; but I have examined the ſerum of the blood of many perſons under inflammatory fevers in this kingdom, but never found it ſo great, ſeldom to exceed ten thouſand three hundred and ſixty-nine, which perhaps may be owing to the air being moiſter here than in England."

That the moiſt ſeaſons in theſe iſlands are remarkably more free from epidemic diſeaſes than the dry ones, appears from the concurrent teſtimonies of the late Engliſh writers on theſe ſubjects, compared to ſimilar obſervations made here; and the ſtorms, the uſual concomitants of rain, are found alſo in both places to be attended with more health and leſs ſickneſs

* Obſervations on the Virtues and Operations of Medicines.

than

than calm weather, as diſſipating the vapours which, by ſtagnation, might prove an occaſion of divers diſeaſes.

Thus, upon a review of the bills of mortality kept in Dublin for forty years, it appears, that the number of perſons buried was remarkably the greateſt in dry years, and vice verſa, v. g.

A. D.	Were buried.
1717	3021
1722	3023
1723	2963
1724	2915
1729	3206
1740	3304

Now in all theſe years drought prevailed: indeed the ſummer of 1724 was wet, but yet otherwiſe fair weather prevailed, as it did in all the reſt of theſe years, particularly and memorably in the years 1723 and 1740, the laſt being the dry year ſucceeding the great froſt, and preſents the greateſt number of all. The years 1704, 1723, and 1740, were eminent for great drought beyond moſt or all others of late obſer-

obſervation, and were accordingly very unhealthy: ſuch ſeaſons, happily for us, are rare; ſo far are we from having cauſe of complaint of our frequent rains.

On the other hand,

A. D.		Were buried.
1730		2184
1734		2466
1735		2196
1743		2193
1744		1705
1746		1957
1754	a wet ſummer	1732
1755	all the ſeaſons wet	1896
1756	ſummer very wet	1550
1758	ſummer rainy	1558

Now each of theſe years was remarkable for a redundant moiſture, except 1743, which was attended with the variable weather proper to the country: but 1744 was

was remarkable for this, that it might be called the year of floods: the year 1746 alſo was a moiſt one, and preſents us with the next leaſt number; and though ſeveral noted perſons died of fevers, yet no general malignity attended them.

Since the year 1746 to 1758, the burials in Dublin have leſſened; however, the far greater part of our ſummers have been wet, and the burials never exceeded two thouſand eighty-eight, but moſtly fell much ſhort of that number.

This is perfectly agreeable to Wintringham's obſervation of the moiſt ſeaſons being more natural and healthful in England, and vice verſa the dry ones, accompanied with eaſterly winds: yet it ſhould ſeem that we are not to underſtand by this but that exceſſive and long continued rains and moiſture are alſo unwholeſome, and productive of diſeaſes, as well as exceſſive drought: for it has appeared upon a review of a long * ſeries

* Short's Chronological Hiſt. of the Weather and Seaſons.

of

of years, that of exceſſive rainy years three out of four were epidemic and mortal, eſpecially when attended with S. or S. W. winds; and that they have this effect, not always primarily, but conſequentially, as they corrupt and ſpoil the fruits of the earth.

It would be perhaps an inſtance of great raſhneſs as well as partiality to the country, to aſſert that no inconveniencies are attendant on the prevailing redundant moiſture and comparative warmth of our air; and that it has no influence on the bodies of the inhabitants, or even in the production and propagation of our endemial diſeaſes.

For we are aſſured †, by good authority, that the inhabitants of wet and damp countries are ſubject to catarrhs and ſeroſities of all kinds, occaſioned by the moiſture of the air imbibed by the pores of the ſkin.

And from this cauſe, and the viciſſitudes of the weather, we may undoubtedly de-

† Langriſh's Mod. Theor. and Practice of Phyſic.

duce

duce the production and propagation of our endemial diseases, viz. defluxions, coughs, tumours of the jaws, and anginas, which make up near three fourths of the catalogue of our prevailing diseases here, as well as at Plymouth *; and it is probable that the stubbornness and fatality of dropsies in this country may also be owing, in a great measure, to the moisture of the climate, as well as the intemperance of the people: wheras Piso †, on the contrary, observes that in Brazil, the operation of the paracentesis is early and happily performed, otherwise than in the northern countries, where their long intemperance has fixed the disease, and Towne observes the same thing in Barbadoes, viz. that the dropsy generally more easily admits of a cure, and the paracentesis is commonly performed with success; and Bontius makes a like remark of the easiness of the cure of the dropsy in the East-Indies.

* Huxham.

† Indiæ utriusq. Hist. Nat. & Med.

A CHRO-

A

CHRONOLOGICAL HISTORY

OF THE

WEATHER, SEASONS, AND DISEASES IN DUBLIN.

SPRING, 1725.

MARCH was moftly fair and pleafant, fometimes fharp and cold: the eleventh high winds at S. E. The principal winds N. E.

April was alternately fair, cloudy, and fhowery. The twentieth and twenty-firft a good deal of rain. The principal winds S. W.

May exhibited a good deal of fair weather, but with clouds and rain interfperfed.

The

The twenty-ſeventh and twenty-eighth ſtormy: the twelfth and twentieth hot, towards the end cold. The principal winds N. E. and S. W. In the ſpring intermitting fevers appeared, which vaniſhed at the beginning of ſummer: alſo ſome exanthematous fevers appeared, which, for for the moſt part, were not dangerous.

SUMMER.

June. Frequent and very plentiful rains, not many fair days, though it concluded fair and very hot. From the ſeventh to the ſeventeenth very cold and unpleaſant. The twenty-third ſtormy and cold. The principal winds W.

July. Rain and cold winds prevailed until the twenty-third, and S. W. winds. The ſeventh and eighth ſtormy.

July. From the twenty-third to the end moſtly fair, ſometimes warm with S. E. and E. winds.

Auguſt. The beginning was moſtly fair, but the remainder was frequently cloudy, wet,

wet, and cold. The ninth, ſixteenth, and twenty-third, much rain, the principal winds W. and S. W. In ſummer there was a purple petechial fever chiefly among the poor, and it was not mortal.

AUTUMN.

September. The firſt half for the moſt part fair, and frequently hot: the latter half there were frequent rains, and it was much colder. The twenty-ſeventh and twenty-eighth much rain and high winds. The principal winds W. and N. E.

October was alternately fair, cloudy, and foggy, with frequent rains: very cold the eighth and tenth. High winds the firſt, twelfth, thirteenth, ſeventeenth, twentieth. The principal winds S. E.

November was fair, cloudy, and wet by intervals; much rain the fifteenth, ſixteenth, and twenty-ninth. High winds the firſt, third, fifteenth, ſixteenth, twenty-fifth and twenty-ninth: the twelfth, thirteenth, and fourteenth, froſty. The principal winds

N. W.

N. W. In September and October a remitting fever was obferved, chiefly among the poor, fometimes attended with purple fpots, and commonly ending with a fweat in fifteen days, and not mortal.

The fum total of burials in Dublin in 1724 was two thoufand nine hundred and forty-one.

WINTER, 1725, 1726.

December. Frofty in the beginning and fome fnow: elfe alternately fair, cloudy, and wet. A ftorm the fecond: high winds the fifth, ninth, twentieth, twenty-firft, and twenty-fecond. The principal winds W.

January was a month of the hardeft weather for fnow, rains, floods, and great inundations over all Europe that ever was known. High winds the firft, fecond, fifteenth, and twenty-feventh. The principal winds N. W. and S. W.

February was cloudy, rarely fair, cold, with frequent fhowers of fnow or fleet. The

The third and ſixth much rain; the eighteenth ſtormy; the twenty-fifth and twenty-ſixth froſty.

SUMMARY.

The ſpring inclined to fair and dry.

The ſummer wet and cold, as over the greateſt part of Europe.

The autumn variable.

A cold winter, ſnow and rain frequent.

SPRING.

March. A good deal of fair weather, though not without clouds and rain; ſome cold, ſome warm days. The twenty-ſecond and thirty-firſt ſtormy. The principal winds S. W.

April. A good deal of fair weather, with ſhowers interſperſed. The thirteenth ſtormy. The principal winds S. W. and N. W.

May. The fair weather of the two preceding months continued, and it was warm; thunder pretty frequent; not much

much rain. The principal winds S. W. and W.

SUMMER.

June. Alternately fair, cloudy, and frequent rains, and ſometimes very hot. The principal winds S. W. and S. E.

July. Fair, but frequent clouds and rain; the two laſt days ſtormy. The principal winds S. W. and N. W.

Auguſt. A good deal of fair weather, and often hot and ſultry, and frequent clouds and rain. The principal winds S. W. and W.

AUTUMN.

September. A prevalence of cloudy and rainy weather; ſome fair days, and concluded fair. The principal winds W.

October. Fair, cloudy, and foggy; little rain: from the eighteenth to the twenty-firſt windy. Winds W. N. W. and S. W.

November. Alternately fair, cloudy, hazy, foggy, and wet; the twelfth ſnow; the

the thirteenth and twenty-fourth ſtormy. The principal winds S. W.

WINTER, 1726, 1727.

December. Moſt of the forepart of the month a hard froſt, and ſometimes hail and ſnow; afterwards alternately fair, cloudy, and wet. The principal winds N. W. and S. W.

January. Alternately fair, cloudy, and wet, and ſometimes a little froſt and ſnow: three ſtormy days. The principal winds S. W.

February. Alternately cloudy, wet, and fair: froſt ſcarce above once or twice. Three ſtormy days. The principal winds E. and S. W.

SUMMARY.

Spring, fair and dry,

Summer, variable.

Autumn, variable.

Winter, for the moſt part open.

In July the cholera morbus was frequent.

The

The ſum total of burials in Dublin 2763.

SPRING.

March. The fore and greater part of the month generally fair and cold: the laſt ten days frequent rains. The principal winds E. S. E. and N. E.

April. Clouds and frequent rains, and ſometimes winds through the month, and ſeveral fair days. The winds moſtly S. E, E. and N. E.

May. Cloudy, and a good deal of rain, eſpecially the latter part of the month, and frequently windy: ſeveral fair and warm days. The principal winds S. E. and E.

SUMMER.

June. Cloudy, rain, and fair weather alternately. The principal winds at ſome point of the E.

July. Frequently cloudy and wet through the month. Several fair days. The principal winds S. E. and S. W

Auguſt. Fair weather generally through the month, except ſome plentiful rains near the

the end. The principal winds N. W. S. E. and S. W.

AUTUMN.

September. Frequently wet and windy through the month; yet many fair days. The principal winds S. W.

October. Rains very frequent through the month; and winds frequent, especially the fore half of it: mizzling fogs, and some fair days the latter part of the month. The principal winds N. W.

November. Alternately fair, cloudy, foggy, and rainy. The principal winds S. W. and N. W.

WINTER, 1727, 1728.

December. Alternately fair, cloudy, foggy, and wet: a little snow and frost. The eleventh and twelfth a storm. The principal wind N. W.

January. Clouds and rain frequent; sometimes foggy, sometimes windy: several fair days. The winds S. E. and S.

February.

February. Fair weather prevailed, but not without clouds, rain, and fogs interpofed. The feventeenth ftormy. The principal winds E. N. W. and W.

SUMMARY.

The fpring variable.

Summer variable, inclined to fair and dry.

Autumn wet.

Winter mild and open.

In April the pleurify was epidemical and mortal in the country, lefs in the city. The fmall-pox this year were very epidemical and mortal.

In November in Staffordfhire and Shropfhire their horfes were fuddenly feized with a cough and weaknefs, difabling them from labour; and in December, both in Dublin, and the remote parts of the kingdom, the horfes were feized with a cough and fhortnefs of breath, and fometimes a forethoat; fome bled at the nofe. A large difcharge of thick phlegm from the nofe, long

long continuing, was falutiferous. Some died in the ftreets, partly through the carelefſnefs of their mafters exercifing them abroad, even during this diforder, partly through neglect of bleeding and purging, and partly from improper medicines.

December 25. The horfes growing better, a cough and fore-throat feized mankind in Dublin. Compare the years 1750 and 1760.

The fum total of burials this year in Dublin, 2946.

SPRING, 1728.

March. Alternately fair, cloudy, wet, and windy. The principal winds W. and N. W.

April. Alternately fair, cloudy, and rainy; and a little wind: fometimes gluts of rain; more frequent the latter part of the month. The principal winds various N. W. S. E. W. S. W. and N. &c.

May.

May. Fair weather prevailed; but clouds and rain frequently interpofed; and fome brifk winds by turns. The principal wind N. W.

In May intermittent fevers were frequent.

SUMMER.

June. Cloudy and a good deal of rain through the month, and brifk winds, efpeally the fore part of the month: feveral fair days. The principal winds W.

July. Alternately fair, cloudy, wet, and fometimes windy. The principal winds N. W. and W.

Auguft. Fair and cloudy weather alternately, and a little rain now and then, and high winds frequent. The principal winds W. N. W. and S. W.

Intermittent fevers mentioned in May, continued in June; and often attacked in the form of a periodical head-ach.

The twenty-third of June ice was found in the river Liffy.

AUTUMN.

AUTUMN.

September. Cloudy, and much rain through the month; ſome fogs, a little windy the fore part of the month. The principal wind E.

October. Alternately fair, cloudy, wet, and ſometimes windy the fore part of the month; the latter part fair and gloomy. Winds N.W. and S.W. the fore part of the month, S.E. and E. the latter part: concluded with a ſtorm at S.W.

November. The fore part of the month cloudy, hazy, frequent rains, and ſome winds; then frequent ſnow, ſleet, hail, and froſt: ended windy and moiſt. The principal wind W.

WINTER, 1728, 1729.

December. Cloudy, wet, ſometimes windy: ſome fair days: froſt and ſnow more ſevere, and of longer duration here and in England than for many years paſt.

The

The principal winds N. N.W. N.E. and S. E.

January. Alternately cloudy, rainy, mizzling, foggy: ſome froſt: windy about the middle of the month. The principal wind W.

February. Cloudy, rainy; a little windy ſometimes: ſeveral ſmart froſts and fair days. The principal winds E. and W.

In December a petechial fever was obſerved; but not mortal; nor was the pulſe quick.

SUMMARY.

The ſpring mild, and for the moſt part fair.

A wet ſummer.

Autumn variable.

Winter variable, inclined to froſt.

SPRING, 1729.

March. Alternately cloudy, hazy, wet, ſometimes windy, ſometimes ſnow, and

ſome

ſome froſt. The principal winds W. and E.

April. Little rain, but moſtly dry and fair, with almoſt a conſtant ſeries of eaſterly winds.

May. Fair weather prevailed, but with rains frequently interſperſed. The wind very variable, moſtly N. W. S. E. and W.

Intermittent fevers were epidemic in April; and ſome of the petechial kind: nor was this altogether peculiar to us: for at that ſame time we were informed that intermittent and other fevers were frequent in the neighbourhood of Glouceſter and London; and very mortal in the country places, but leſs in the cities.

SUMMER.

June. Cloudy and frequent rains through the month; and fair days alſo pretty frequently interſperſed. The principal winds W. S. E. E. and S. W.

July.

July. The firſt twelve days moſtly fair and dry, and a ſeries of Eaſterly winds for the moſt part: the reſt of the month W. and N. W. with frequent rains, and ſeveral fair days interpoſed.

Auguſt. Except the beginning and near the end, when there were frequent rains, the middle and greater part of the month was fair. The principal wind E.

AUTUMN.

September wet and windy, eſpecially the latter part of the month, but many fair days. The principal winds S. E. E. S. and W.

October alternately cloudy, hazy, rain, and fair weather, and ſometimes windy. The principal winds W.

November. A month of much rain, and ſtormy: very few fair days. The principal winds W. N. W. and S.

From Auguſt to October a petechial fever appeared, in which the primæ viæ and head were much affected: it ſeldom

proved

proved mortal, and vaniſhed without ſenſible evacuation, the urine continuing crude, with a languid motion of the blood.

In November raged an univerſal epidemic catarrh, ſcarce ſparing any one family, being attended with a cough, soreneſs of the breaſt, with ſome pain of the head and back, and a ſlight fever. It was common to us and London, Dorſetſhire, &c. and proved fatal chiefly to old perſons. It viſited London before us, where, in the beginning of the month, there died nine hundred, and by November the eighteenth, a thouſand, which is ſaid to be more than have died in that city in the ſame ſpace of time ſince the year 1665.

In Dublin, December the thirteenth, the weekly bill amounted to one hundred and eighteen, near double the uſual number. It is ſaid that the like epidemic prevailed over great part of Europe this year.

Compare the years 1732-33, 1737, and 1743.

WIN-

WINTER, 1729, 1730.

December much rain and winds, and this diſpoſition ſeems to have prevailed elſewhere; for there were great floods in England and in Italy: often foggy and hazy. The principal winds W. S. W. and S. E.

January fair, hazy and foggy: little rain: high winds the twenty-ſecond, twenty-eighth, twenty-ninth. The thirty-firſt froſt, being the firſt hard weather this winter. The principal wind W.

February much rain, and frequent high winds; at the latter end froſt and ſnow. The principal wind W.

SUMMARY.

A cold and dry ſpring.

A dry ſummer moſtly.

Autumn inclined to wet and windy.

Winter open, much rain, and ſomewhat windy.

The

The ſum total of burials this year three thouſand two hundred and ſix, a large number, to which the epidemic catarrh contributed.

SPRING, 1730.

March. Much rain: a few fair days. The ſeventh, eleventh, and twelfth, windy. The principal winds W. and N. W.

April. The firſt half, and great part of the month, was frequently cloudy and wet; the eleventh and twelfth windy, and the principal winds N. W. but from the eighteenth to the end it was fair, and the principal wind E.

May. The dry weather, with E. and N. E. winds, continued to the tenth day; after which there were not many days free from rain. The twenty-ninth and thirtieth windy. The principal winds E. W. and S.

SUM-

SUMMER.

June. Cloudy, rainy, and cold weather prevailed : windy for the fore-part of the month. The principal winds W. N. N. W. and E.

July. Cloudy and wet weather ſtill prevailed : few fair days. The firſt, ſecond, and twenty-ninth windy. The principal winds N. W. and W.

Auguſt. Fair and dry weather prevailed, though hazy, cloudy, and wet by turns. The principal winds S. W. E. and W.

Intermittent fevers were frequent in May, as they were alſo in ſummer, both here and in London, and elſewhere in England, and often obſtinate.

AUTUMN.

September. Fair weather prevailed : the tenth remarkably cold, cloudy, and wet, between whiles. The twentieth, twenty-

firſt,

firſt, and twenty-ſecond a damp fog. The principal wind W.

October, excepting a few fair and ſome hazy days, cloudy and rainy weather prevailed, and it was windy near the end. The principal winds W. and S. E.

November alternately foggy, wet, cloudy, and fair, ſometimes windy: the laſt week froſt. The principal wind W.

WINTER, 1730, 1731.

December many fair days, ſome cloudy, hazy and foggy: rain frequent. The ninth windy. The principal winds W. and N. W.

January. The beginning of the month variable: from the ninth to the twenty-third moſtly fair, ſometimes hazy and foggy: near the end more wet, with ſnow and ſleet. The principal wind W.

February cloudy and wet through great part of the month, the ninth a great ſtorm: the ſecond a hard froſt. The principal winds S. S. W. and W.

SUM-

SUMMARY.

The ſpring variable.

Summer wet.

Autumn variable.

Winter open, mild, and comparatively dry.

The ſum total of burials this year two thouſand one hundred and eighty-four.

SPRING, 1731.

March. Uncommonly ſerene, calm, and dry. The principal winds W. S. W. and N. W. The month concluded with S. E. and E. winds.

April. An unuſually dry and cold month for the moſt part: a little ſnow. The fifteenth, ſixteenth, and twenty-fifth, rainy. The principal winds S. E. N. E, and E.

May. The cold weather continued to the thirteenth day. The firſt nineteen days alternities of fair, cloudy, and wet weather;

weather: from the twentieth to the end moſtly fair and hot. The principal wind W.

The dryneſs and coldneſs of the fore-part of the ſpring was common to us and other parts, particularly to the Baltick, to Hamburgh, and to ſome parts of France.

SUMMER.

June. Dry and frequently ſultry, though with cloudy, hazy, and a little wet weather interſperſed. The principal wind W.

July. Generally ſerene, dry, and frequently very hot, yet rain often interſperſed. The principal wind W.

Auguſt. Generally fair, and frequently hot. The twenty-third, twenty-fourth, twenty-fifth, and twenty-ſixth rainy; moſtly from the S. E. which was the principal wind of the month.

Doctors Rogers and Connel agree, that in the years 1727, 1728, 1729, 1730,

1731,

1731, the reigning fevers in Cork were for the moſt part of the low kind, in which the pulſe was commonly depreſſed; and they generally did not bear bleeding, and reigned in winter as well as ſummer, and are called by Rogers the endemial epidemics of Cork; but this kind of fever at the time above mentioned was far from being peculiar to Cork, and therefore muſt have been owing not to the particular ſituation of that city, but to ſome more extenſive cauſe common to it and other places: for upon a review of the reigning weather and diſeaſes in Dublin at the ſame time, viz. 1727, 1728, 1729, 1730, I find that the general diſpoſition of the weather in both places was to a redundance of moiſture: the winters were open, there was very little froſt, and the ſummer in 1730 was very wet: and I find that during the ſame time the reigning fever in Dublin was preciſely of the ſame kind; mild and deceitful in its firſt attack, attended with

a

a depreſſed pulſe, and frequently with petechiæ.

In Auguſt and September diarrhœas were frequent.

AUTUMN.

September, Fair weather prevailed: ſeveral warm days; yet frequent rains, and windy at the beginning and end. The principal wind W.

October. Variable, cloudy, and frequent rains, fair, mizzling, hazy, and foggy alternately, and ſometimes a little windy. Winds S. W. and S. E.

November. Cloudy and wet weather prevailed, and ſometimes windy: the twenty-ſixth a froſt. The principal wind W.

WINTER. 1731, 1732.

December. Cloudy, moiſt, and rainy weather prevailed: windy ſometimes. Froſt and ſnow the latter part of the month. The principal wind W.

Janu-

January. Generally cloudy and wet; but a few fair days. The laſt two weeks warm. The principal wind S. E.

February. Cloudy, wet, windy, and unuſually warm this month. The principal wind W.

SUMMARY.

A dry and cold ſpring, but concluded hot.

A hot and dry ſummer.

Autumn variable, and ſometimes windy.

Winter wet and warm.

The ſum total of burials this year 2184.

SPRING 1732.

March. Windy at the beginning, then alternities of fair, cloudy, and wet weather. The tenth and eleventh ſnow, the twenty-ſixth hail: the three laſt days plentiful rain. The principal winds N. W.

April. Alternities of fair and cloudy weather, and ſhowers. The fourteenth and

twenty-

twenty-ninth hail. The principal winds N. S. E. N. E. S. W.

May. Cloudy and rainy weather prevailed, but a few fair days. The principal winds S.W. S. S. E. and E.

In the three ſpring months coughs, and a few peripneumonies, and aguiſh diſorders occurred, which laſt were alſo epidemic in the country at the ſame time.

SUMMER.

June. Fair weather for the moſt part, but a little rain. The principal winds W. N.W. E. and S. E.

July. Cloudy and rainy weather prevailed; ſometimes a little windy, ſeveral ſultry days, and ſome cold. The principal winds W. N. W. and S. W.

Auguſt. Fair weather prevailed. The twelfth and thirteenth much rain: the twenty-fifth and twenty-ſixth windy. The principal winds W. and E.

A U-

AUTUMN.

September. The firſt nine days generally fair, the reſt of the month for the moſt part windy, cloudy, and wet. The principal winds S. E. and W.

October. Cloudy, wet, and windy weather prevailed. The principal wind W.

November. Fair, gloomy, ſometimes foggy: frequently froſty: little rain or wind. The principal winds N. and N. W.

Some agues appeared in autumn, both in the town and country, which did not wholly diſappear in the winter.

I did not learn that there had been any thing epidemic this ſummer or autumn; the few fevers that I met with in both thoſe ſeaſons were of the low kind.

WINTER, 1732, 1733.

December. The greateſt part of the firſt thirteen days fair, the remainder clou-

cloudy, wet, and windy: a very warm Chriſtmas. A great ſtorm the twentieth at night, and the twenty-firſt at W. Another the twenty-ninth and thirtieth at S. W. and W. The principal winds S. E. W. and S. W.

January. Cloudy, wet, windy, and unſeaſonably warm: a few fair days: the fourth a ſtorm at S. and S. W. the ſeventh another at S.W. the twenty-ninth another at S. W. The principal winds S. W.

February. Cloudy, wet, and ſtormy weather continued through the month: ſcarce one entire fair day, viz. the ninth. The firſt a ſtorm at S. W. The third and fourth another at W. and S. W. The nineteenth another. The principal winds W. S. W. and N. W.

SUMMARY.

Variable weather in the ſpring, the laſt month rainy.

Summer moderately fair and dry.

Autumn wet and windy.

A wet

A wet, windy, ſtormy, and warm winter.

The cloſe of the year exhibited a remarkable epidemic, of foreign original, and like that above deſcribed in 1729, but more mortal, as the ſeaſon was more advanced, viz. a catarrhal fever, or fever of cold, having previouſly viſited Germany and Great Britain, and ſpread itſelf afterwards, not only over moſt parts of Europe, but travelled even to America, being perhaps the moſt univerſal diſeaſe upon record.

It began at Edinburgh December ſeventeenth, became very epidemic the twenty-fifth, until the middle of January, when it began to decreaſe, and diminiſhed daily till the end of that month. See vol. ii. *Edinburgh Medical Eſſays*; where it is alſo obſerved that the horſes were univerſally attacked with a running of the noſe and cough towards the end of October and beginning of November before the appearance of this catarrhal fever among men.

It

It made its appearance in Dublin about the end of January, and continued throughout the month of February, and the weekly bills of mortality at their greateſt height were 169, being about treble their uſual ſtandard; and in London at the height of this epidemical diſorder their bills amounted to 1588, viz. a greater number than for ſeventy years before.

Very few eſcaped it here. It was introduced by an acute fever, but of ſhort duration, commonly ending in a running of the noſe and eyes, more rarely a cough. A ſpontaneous ſweating commonly attended, and relieved, and appeared to be the natural criſis, though bleeding and purging were frequently practiſed with ſucceſs, and the blood drawn was obſerved to be ſizy.

It proved mortal to few and thoſe chiefly children, and aſthmatic and conſumptive old men; and herein it remarkably differed from the *ſudor Anglicus*, to whch children and old people were leſs ſubject.

Dr.

Dr. Short's obſervation in his Cronological Hiſtory of the Weather and Seaſons, may deſerve attention, viz. that bleeding was chiefly ſerviceable to thoſe who had a pain or weight at the breaſt, and that whilſt the fever was coming on, not going off: for in the laſt caſe it hurted, and left a bad cough and weakneſs.

N. B. The Dunkirk fever, ſo called from its being brought by our ſoldiers from that place, and which Dr. Mead reckons a ſpecies of the *ſudor Anglicus*, which viſited London in 1713, viſited us here alſo, and was mortal to few.

The author mentioned deduces its original from the plague, which a few years before broke out at Dantzic. At London it began only with a pain in the head, and went off in large ſweats, uſually after a day's confinement; but at Dunkirk it was attended with the additional ſymptoms of vomiting, diarrhœa, &c. See *Mead* of the Plague.

The

The ſum total of burials this year in Dublin was two thouſand five hundred thirty-four.

SPRING, 1733.

March. Alternities of cloudy and fair weather at the beginning; but the ſucceeding and greater part of the month frequent ſnows, rains, and ſleet, and exceſſively cold. The twenty-fifth very warm, and concluded warm and fair. The winds N. E. S. E. N. W. and N.

April. Fair and dry weather prevailed, though variegated with clouds and rain. The principal winds E. N. E. and S. E.

May. Uncommonly fair and dry through the greateſt part of the month. The principal winds S. E. E. and N. E.

SUMMER.

June. Fair and dry the firſt ſix days: afterwards ſhowers were interſperſed; though fair weather prevailed through the month in general. The thirteenth and twenty-

twenty-eighth thunder. The principal wind S. E.

July. Fair and dry for the moft part. The fifth, fixth, and feventh, hot and fultry; the fixteenth and feventeenth thunder, lightning, and rain. The principal winds W. and N.W.

Auguft. Cloudy, and frequently wet and windy: a cold month and a fudden onfet as of winter. The twelfth a ftorm at W. The principal winds W. N.W. and S.W.

AUTUMN.

September. Some fair days, but for the moft part cloudy, wet, and windy. The twenty-fixth thunder. The principal winds N. W. and S. E.

October. Moftly fair: windy towards the end. The twentieth a hoar-froft. The principal winds S. W. S. E. and N.

November. For the moft part cloudy, wet, and windy. The principal winds S.W. and W.

WIN-

WINTER, 1733, 1734.

December. Wet and very windy. The eleventh, twelfth, thirteenth, and fourteenth, ſtormy at S.W. the thirteenth thunder and hail : the twenty-third high wind at S.W. with lightning, like a whirlwind or tornado. The principal winds S. W. and S.

January. The firſt ſeven days ſome ſnow and froſt, and this partly with a S. W. wind : alſo the thirteenth and fourteenth froſt : the ninth and tenth rainy : the reſt of the month for the moſt part fair, and ſometimes cloudy, foggy, and hazy : winds various, W. S. W. S. E. and N. W.

February. The firſt half of the month generally fair and dry, the remaining part moſtly cloudy, wet, and windy ; the twelfth warm, the fourteenth and fifteenth a ſtorm, and continued windy the three following days. The principal winds W. S.W. and S.

SUM-

SUMMARY.

A very dry ſpring.

A dry ſummer, but ended wet and windy.

A wet and windy autumn.

A wet, windy, and very warm winter, and ſo in England. The primroſes and violets were bloſſoming at Chriſtmas.

Some agues and intermitting diſorders and anginas occurred in the ſpring; but in ſummer the agues became very epidemic, and continued in autumn; when alſo a few ſporadic, low, petechial fevers appeared, and ſeveral diarrhœas and dyſenteries in autumn and in December.

Perhaps the dryneſs of the ſpring, and part of the ſummer, may be here obſerved as no way favouring the common ſuppoſition of the aguiſh conſtitution being promoted by the contrary diſpoſition of the air, viz. redundant moiſture, which was remarkably the caſe in the two following years.

To

To this I anſwer, Firſt, that in accounting for the operation of the weather on human bodies, we are to attend not only to the preſent prevailing ſtate of the air, but alſo to the preceding condition of it; which ſometimes may not operate until ſucceeded by a contrary temperature. Now in the preſent caſe, it is certain that the preceding winter was exceſſively moiſt and warm, and even the preceding autumn was wet and windy: and as the petechial fever which attended the moiſt winters of 1734 and 1735, became more epidemic in the ſubſequent hot ſummer of 1736, and as ſome inflammatory diſorders, which owed their origin to the intenſeneſs of the cold as a prediſpoſing cauſe, have been obſerved to become more frequent on the thaw, why might not the like viciſſitude have an analogous effect in the preſent caſe?

Secondly, Different diſeaſes may attend the ſame ſtate of the weather from the difference of the conſtitutions of men, which

which Dr. Huxham has ingenioufly accounted for in his Effay on Fevers in the following words: " Sometimes intermitting fevers are very rife and contemporary with epidemic pleurifies and peripneumonies, as was particularly obferved in the year 1744; and this diverfity of effects from the cold air may eafily be deduced from the diverfity of conftitutions; viz. in fome bracing up the fibres and infpiffating the humours to that degree of vifcidity as to produce inflammatory fevers; whilft in others of a laxer habit, it only produced fuch a degree of vifcidity as is proper to intermittents."

Thirdly, According to Dr. Short's obfervation in his Chronological Hiftory of the Weather and Seafons, on a review of thefe for feveral centuries, it appears, that agues attend any exceffes of the feafons, whether the exceffively droughty and hot, or the exceffively wet and rainy; and that they are alfo the product of inequalities of the feafons, agreeably to the above obfervations

vations cited from the German Ephemerides, v. g. of uncommon heat immediately ſucceeding ſevere cold, or intenſe cold ſucceeding great heat.

The ſum total of burials this year was two thouſand ſix hundred and eight.

SPRING, 1734.

March. Wet and windy: the twenty-third a ſtorm at S. The principal winds S. W. and W.

April. Warm and ſerene like June, eſpecially to the ſixteenth day, and a forward ſpring: the latter part of the month ſhowers more frequent, and ſometimes a little hail: the nineteenth, cold and a ſtorm at night, with lightning. The principal winds S. E. and S. W.

May. Unuſually cold, with alternities of fair, cloudy, and wet weather, but frequently hail, ſome hoar-froſts and ſnow; ſo that the twenty-fourth was the firſt ſummer-like day. The fourteenth and fifteenth hail, thunder, and lightning: the

the twenty-ſixth, twenty-ſeventh, twenty-eighth, a great fall of rain with N. E. and S. E. winds. The principal winds N. N. W. S. E. and E.

In the ſpring appeared ſome agues and coughs.

SUMMER.

June. Cloudy and wet weather prevailed. The principal winds S. E.

July. Cloudy, wet, and mizzling weather prevailed. The principal wind W.

Auguſt. Fair weather prevailed, but clouds and ſhowers were frequently interſperſed: the latter part of the month windy. The principal winds W. and S. E.

In the ſummer agues were frequent.

AUTUMN.

September. The beginning and end of the month wet and windy, the middle moſtly fair. The principal winds W. and S. W.

October.

October. The firſt day a ſtorm at S. W. and thunder and lightning: elſe ſerene, cloudy, hazy, foggy, mizzling and rain alternately. The principal winds S. W. N. W. and W.

November. Alternities of fair, cloudy, hazy, and foggy weather: the eighth and twenty-ſeventh froſt, twenty-fifth and twenty-ſixth ſnow, twenty-eighth and twenty-ninth ſtormy at W. and S. W. twenty-third and twenty-fourth rainy. The principal wind S. E.

WINTER, 1734, 1735.

December. Cloudy, rainy, and windy weather prevailed: a few fair days: the fourteenth a great ſtorm at S. W. the twenty-ſecond froſt. The principal winds W. S. W. and N. W.

January. Cloudy, rainy and windy weather prevailed; ſometimes foggy and mizzling. The ſeventh and eighth a ſtorm at S. W. the ninth, tenth, fourteenth, fifteenth, twenty-firſt and twenty-fifth froſt.

The

The principal winds W. S. W. and N. W.

February. Cloudy, mizzling, and moiſt for the moſt part to the ſeventeenth: the ſixth warm like ſummer: from the ſeventeenth to the end fairer: the nineteenth ſnow and hail: the twenty-firſt froſt. The ſeventh, tenth, and twenty-third windy at S. W. and W. the principal winds S. W. W. and N. W.

SUMMARY.

The two firſt months of ſpring very warm (and ſo in England) but followed by a cold and nipping May, which hurted the fruits, and burnt the graſs.

A wet ſummer: much ſtraw and little grain: graſs plentiful in the uplands.

Autumn variable.

A wet, windy, and generally mild winter.

N. B. The ſtate of the weather in England from Short's Chronological Hiſtory of the Weather and Seaſons, agrees very

very nearly to ours, viz. " From September the twenty-eighth 1731, to June the twelfth 1734, it was moſtly droughty, no general or great floods or rains, and the ſprings failed in moſt places: then June the twelfth 1734, began the long wet ſeaſon, and continued moſtly to February the ſecond 1736, viz. a year and eight months, after two years and nine months drought."

In autumn (and eſpecially in winter, when alſo ſome agues appeared) we had the low fever called nervous (and ſometimes petechial from the ſpots that frequently attended, altho' probably not eſſential) the diſtinguiſhing ſymptoms of which were chiefly, that the firſt attack was frequently ſlow and deceitful, the pulſe ſometimes ſcarce quicker than in health, elſe quick and low, nor was the heat great or conſtant: they had frequent ſuſpiria or laborious breathing.

The time of the criſis was various, as the ſeventh, eleventh, fifteenth, and one

and

and twentieth days. I obſerved ſeveral of theſe to recover eaſily.

It is no new thing with us for this low kind of fever to prevail in the winter ſeaſon: for it did ſo likewiſe in the ſame ſeaſon in the morbid conſtitution of 1727, 1728, 1729, and 1730; as alſo in 1735, and in the years 1745 and 1746.

And it may be worth obſerving that this diſorder is far from being peculiar to theſe iſlands: for I find in the epidemic conſtitutions in Germany, that the petechial and purple ſpotted fever, wherein the quickneſs of the pulſe and heat of the body was ſcarce greater than in health, did as frequently attend on a changeable ſtate of weather in winter, as much or rather more than in other ſeaſons of the year; and moreover I find by a medium taken by Dr. Bryan Robinſon, of the number of deaths each quarter for forty years, from the bills of mortality in Dublin, that the greateſt number from fever actually happened in the winter-quarter; ſo that,

altho'

altho' the number of deaths from the article of fever in the summer-quarter was greater than either in ſpring or autumn, yet it was leſs than in winter, viz. as ſeventeen thouſand five hundred and twenty-three, to eighteen thouſand two hundred and eighty.

It is moreover obſervable, that this and the following year were not leſs remarkable for extraordinary moiſture, than for the prevalence of the ſame epidemic diſeaſes, viz. chiefly the intermittent and low kind of fevers. The ſum total of the burials this year was two thouſand four hundred and ſixty-ſix.

SPRING 1735.

March. Cloudy and wet weather prevailed. The thirteenth, nineteenth, twentieth, and twenty-fourth cold, and ſome froſt, ſnow, or hail. The principal winds N.E. S.E. and N.W.

April was alternately fair, cloudy, and wet as uſual. The principal winds S.E. W. N.E. and S.W.

May

May was cold, dry, and parching, ſometimes cloudy and a little wet, ſometimes hail. The principal winds N.W. N. N. E.

SUMMER.

June. Cloudy, wet, and cold weather prevailed, ſometimes windy. The principal winds W. S.W. and N.W.

July was cloudy, wet, and cold, ſometimes windy, few ſummer days. A very backward ſeaſon in fruits and grain. The principal winds N.W. S.E. S.W. and W.

Auguſt. The firſt eleven days generally fair, and the winds S.E. and N.E. thence to the end wet and windy with S.W. and W. winds.

Hear Dr. Huxham's melancholic deſcription of their ſummer this year at Plymouth, having been much like ours, viz. "Omnes fructus horæi acerbi ſunt & immaturi : vix audis cicadam : rari volitant papiliones : plurimæ aviculæ canentes inter plumas exuendas intereunt."

Agues,

Agues, which had been frequent in April and May, were protracted to June and July, and required the utmoſt attention and ſagacity in the phyſician, being frequently diſguiſed under the appearance of other diſeaſes; and thoſe who were attacked with them, were ſubject to frequent relapſes: and Huxham makes the like obſervation of the agues at Plymouth in the years 1734 and 1735, viz. that even the vernal tertians were very obſtinate, and the patients ſubject to relapſes on the ſlighteſt occaſions. At the latter end of May and beginning of June, ſlight anginas prevailed much.

In June and July appeared ſome ſporadic petechial fevers; but we ſhall ſee that theſe grow more frequent at the latter end of winter.

AUTUMN.

September was for the moſt part cloudy and rainy, ſometimes windy; the two firſt days very ſultry, cold afterwards: the

the twentieth hot again. The principal winds S.E. and W.

October was hazy and cloudy, with frequent rains, yet ſeveral fair days. The firſt, eleventh, twenty-eighth, and thirtieth cold. The principal winds S. E. and E.

November. Wet and windy weather prevailed, there were but few fair days. The principal winds S.E. W. S.W. and N.W.

In autumn the intermittent fevers or agues were obſerved remarkably to affect the ſtomach and bowels with a tendency to a diarrhœa, which laſt diſorder alſo, without a fever, prevailed much about the ſame time.

WINTER, 1735, 1736.

December. Cloudy, wet, and mizzling weather prevailed. The eighth thunder and lightning; the fifth, fourteenth, and fifteenth froſt. The principal winds S.E. S.W. and W.

On

On Chriſtmas-day ſome pear-trees were in bloſſom.

January was very rainy and frequently windy: the fourteenth, fifteenth, ſixteenth, and twenty-third froſt, ſome little ſnow and ſleet interſperſed: the principal winds S.W. and S.E. both attended with wet weather.

February. A good deal of rain, and frequently ſnow and ſleet, the twelfth, eighteenth, and twenty-fourth froſt. The principal winds N.W. N. S.E. and E.

SUMMARY.

Of the ſpring the two firſt months were pretty open; but ſucceeded by a cold and dry May.

The ſummer cold and wet like winter.

Autumn wet.

Winter open.

Abundance of moiſture thro' the three ſeaſons of ſummer, autumn, and winter.

In December and January there was a fever, which in divers ſubjects agreed in many

many common ſymptoms, and particularly in the ſupervening event of rheumatic pains ſucceeding in thoſe who ſurvived. Towards the eighth of January ſomething like this became epidemical, at leaſt in the barracks, reſembling a true pleuriſy, as to pain, fever, pulſe, and ſizy blood, in which bleeding was ordered and repeated; tho' it was obſervable that moſt that were bled died: but thoſe in whom bleeding was omitted recovered, and in theſe it commonly ended in a rheumatic pain in the ſhoulder, as the ſide became diſengaged.

This may ſerve as an inſtance of the importance of Wintringham's obſervation in his Commentarium Noſologicum, viz. that it is of uſe to attend to the qualities of the ſeaſons accompanying epidemic diſeaſes, inſomuch that in a hot and dry intemperature of the air long continuing, the degree of inflammation and other ſymptoms depending thereon, are more violent, and even ſo far as to require a different

treat-

treatment, v. g. more bleeding, but in a cold and moiſt intemperature of the air (which was egregiouſly the caſe here) the blood was leſs inflamed, and leſs bleeding was required: and to this agrees Huxham's remark, that in continued wet weather, perſons under pleuritic diſorders, in general, do not bear the loſs of much blood.

Towards the end of January and in February, petechial fevers were frequent, and fatal to ſeveral, notwithſtanding the repeated application of bliſters, and the liberal uſe of ſtrong cordials.

There was alſo this winter-quarter, at the ſame time with the petechial, a fever attended with a diarrhœa, almoſt through the whole courſe of it, with great weakneſs, the tongue white, but ſeldom dry: for many days before the fever ceaſed, they made large quantities of an almoſt limpid urine.

Plentiful diluting with decoctum album, the uſe of the teſtacea and rhu-

barb,

barb, with diaſcordium, ſucceeded beſt: this fever laſted ſometimes above twenty days.

It is very obvious to ſuppoſe, that ſuch a conſtitution of the air, as the above deſcribed, which was neither able to bring fruits to maturity, nor to invigorate and enliven other animals, did alſo greatly relax and leave unſtrung the fibres conſtituting the vaſcular ſyſtem in the human body; and, conſequently, was leſs able to bring fevers to a ſpeedy coction by ſweat, their moſt frequent and natural criſis.

To this agrees Aph. 16. lib. 3. of Hippocrates. "Aſſiduis imbribus morbi fere fiunt febres longæ, fluxiones alvi, putredines, prolapſus cartilaginis, enſiformis, &c." And Short, in his Chronological Hiſtory of the Weather and Seaſons, remarks as a frequent thing, that in a moiſt, ſoutherly, rainy ſeaſon, a looſeneſs attends the diſeaſes of the conſtitution.

This, viz. the petechial fever, was frequent, not only here, but in England and

Scotland

Scotland this year, and attacked chiefly the poorer ſort, not wine-drinkers. See MED. ESSAYS, vol. 4.

Short, on a ſurvey of a long ſeries of the prevailing concomitant weather and diſeaſes, obſerves, that the far greater part of the epidemic ſeaſons of ſpotted fevers, were from rain, or from moiſt and ſoutherly conſtitutions.

March. Alternately fair and cloudy the firſt ten days, and cold and ſnow ſometimes; thence to the eighteenth, fair and ſummer-like; thence to the end, often cloudy and wet. The principal winds S. E. S. N. E. and E.

April. Alternately fair, cloudy, and rainy: from the tenth to the fifteenth cold, and hail and froſt. The principal winds S. E. and N. W.

May fair, but frequent and plentiful rains were interpoſed: the nineteenth and thirty-firſt days very hot, the principal winds S. E. and N. E.

Pete-

Petechial fevers, which had been frequent laſt winter, continued to be ſo in March, nor was April and May free from them.

April was the moſt unhealthy of the three ſpring months: throughout this month were frequent, certain eruptions on the ſkin called raſhes, affecting chiefly young perſons, in ſome meaſure reſembling the meazles, but wanting the pathognomonic ſigns. Some feveriſhneſs commonly preceded the eruption: they commonly vaniſhed in forty-eight hours, nor required the aſſiſtance of the phyſician.

There appeared alſo in the ſame month ſome intermitting diſorders, but irregular in their type, and ſome violent colds, almoſt equal to fevers, though not confining the perſons affected to their beds.

SUMMER.

June. Moſtly fair and very hot, the hotteſt June that is remembered ſince the year

year 1723. The principal winds E. S. E. N. E. W. and N. W.

July. Moſtly fair and hot, but not without ſhowers. The principal winds W. S. W. S. E. S. E. and N. E.

Auguſt. Fair weather prevailed, but clouds and rain frequently interpoſed. The principal winds S. E. S. W. and N. W.

This ſummer was as remarkable for heat, as the preceding one had been for coldneſs and moiſture. Such tranſitions from one extreme to another muſt undoubtedly affect the human body; and, according to the concurrent obſervations of Wintringham and Huxham, prediſpoſe to the petechial fevers which attended, and became much more frequent and fatal to ſeveral (eſpecially to thoſe of higher condition) being advanced to a higher degree of malignity by the exceſſive heat of the ſeaſon*, and accordingly, there was the

* It has been obſerved of ſpotted fevers, that though they may ſet in at all times of the year, yet, like the plague, they generally diſplay their fatal virulence at ſummer and harveſt.

greateſt

greateſt increaſe of deaths in the weekly bills during ſummer, and chiefly by the articles of fever and ſmall pox.

The principal diſtinguiſhing ſymptoms of the aforeſaid fever were an anxiety, frequent ſighing, a heavy and laborious breathing, a delirium, and ſubſultus tendinum; and theſe ſymptoms, increaſed with a ſupervening coma, uſually put an end to the tragical ſcene. The pulſe was various; for though it was frequently low and weak, it was ſometimes ſtrong and full, as divers authors have obſerved the pulſe to be weak and low in the beginning, but to become ſtronger in the progreſs of the low nervous fevers; the blood not always florid, but ſizy in ſome. The ſpots obſerved no certain time in their eruption, nor agreed in their dimenſions nor colour, which in different ſubjects was diverſified through all the ſeveral ſhades from a red to a purple.

It proved fatal to ſome the tenth or eleventh, to others the fourteenth, to

ſome

ſome the twenty-firſt or twenty-fourth day. A bilious diarrhœa frequently attended, which it was dangerous either to reſtrain ſuddenly, or to let run too long; for in the firſt caſe worſe ſymptoms followed; in the latter, the criſis (which when left to nature was often by ſweat) was protracted.

As to the uſe of bliſters, though I know that ſeveral emerged on their application, and believe that under ſome circumſtances they might have been properly applied, yet it muſt be acknowledged that they more frequently proved unſucceſsful, even in the hands of the learned, among perſons of note; whilſt many of the poor, with a diet entirely low, and chiefly the uſe of their uſual julep, butter-milk-whey, and with little or no medicines, recovered; which, whether it was owing to the want of a due attention to Baglivi's caution againſt the uſe of the cantharides in hot and dry habits of body, in very hot weather, and where the blood inclines to a

colli-

colliquative ſtate, or whether this diverſity of the fate of the rich and poor were owing to a more putreſcent ſtate of the animal juices, promoted by the freer uſe of animal food among the former than among the latter, or to the invincible difficulty of the caſes, when the phyſician has the misfortune (as he too often has) of being called in when nature is ſinking under her laſt ſtruggles, I ſhall leave to be determined by others upon mature deliberation.

AUTUMN.

September ſerene, but frequently cloudy, foggy, mizzling, and ſometimes a little rain and wind. The principal winds S. W. N. W. and W.

October. Fair weather prevailed, cloudy, foggy, and wet at intervals. The twenty-fifth and twenty-ſixth an unuſual warmth in the air, followed by great ſtorms at S. W. the twenty-ſeventh, twenty-eighth, twenty-ninth, and thirtieth. The principal winds S. W. W. and S. E.

No-

November. Fair, but with frequent clouds, ſome fogs and rain, and often windy. The twenty-ſixth and twenty-ſeventh a froſt. The principal winds W. and N. W.

From the latter end of Auguſt, and throughout September, appeared a few intermittent fevers, and very irregular, but the fever of laſt ſummer was much rarer. The fore part of September exhibited, as uſual, ſeveral diarrhœas and dyſenteries, and October ſome choleras.

WINTER, 1736, 1737.

December. Wet and windy for the moſt part, but a few fair days: the fourteenth ſnow: the fifteenth and twenty-firſt froſty. The principal winds W. and S. W.

January. Cloudy, hazy, and frequently wet and windy, but a few fair days. The principal winds W. and N. W. January the ſeventeenth, a ſpring of graſs appeared in the country.

Fe-

February. Cloudy, windy, and wet: a few fair days. The thirteenth a ſtorm at S. W. The ſixteenth and ſeventeenth, another at S. W. and W. The principal winds N. W. W. and S. W.

SUMMARY.

A mild ſpring for the moſt part, though not without ſome froſt and changeable weather.

One of the hotteſt ſummers that has been remembered.

Autumn moderately fair and mild. Winter very open, wet, and windy: little froſt.

The three winter months exhibited ſcarce any thing remarkable but colds, which were common to us and ſome parts of England at the ſame time, particularly in January, when there was a very epidemic one, ſcarce ſparing a family: it was violent in its attack, yet by keeping warm and diluting, it vaniſhed in a few days; but if neglected in the beginning, it put on the

the appearance of a peripneumonia notha, with great cough, and in many, eryſipelatous ſwellings in the face.

The ſum total of burials this year was two thouſand one hundred and one.

SPRING, 1737.

March. Variable from ſerene to cloudy, and rain interſperſed. The principal winds S. E. N. W. and W.

April. Fair, cloudy, rain and ſqually weather interchangeably, but fair weather prevailed. The principal winds E. S. E. N. E. and S. W.

May. The fore part of the month fair, cloudy, and a little rain alternately; the latter part hot and dry. The principal winds throughout the month S. E. and E.

SUMMER.

June. Fair weather prevailed, ſometimes cloudy and a little rain: ſeveral cold days the fore part of the month, and hot ones

ones the latter part. The principal winds N. W. W. S. E. N. E. and E.

July. Generally fair, except ſome ſhowers at the latter end. The firſt nine days exceſſively hot. The twenty-firſt a ſtorm at S. W. winds variable S. W. N. W. E. S. E. and N. E.

Auguſt. Cloudy, wet, windy, and cold weather prevailed. The ſixth a ſlight froſt. The dog-days cold both in England and Ireland. The principal winds N. W. S. W. and N.

AUTUMN.

September. Fair weather prevailed; ſome days ſultry like dog-days: ſome clouds and rain interſperſed. The principal winds S. E. S. W. N. W. and W.

October. Fair weather prevailed, but clouds and rain were frequently interpoſed. The principal winds N. E. N. S. W. S. E. and E.

November. As in the two preceding months, the fair weather rather prevailed, but

but with alternities of cloudy, windy, mizzling weather, and rain. The twenty-ninth a froſt. The principal winds W. and S. W.

(I ſpent good part of the ſummer this year in England; but Dr. Richard Weld continued the Diary of the Weather in Dublin during my abſence; and as to the diſeaſes I can only give what ſeemed moſt remarkable in autumn and winter.)

Some dyſenteries appeared in Auguſt and September; and in the beginning of September ſeveral chin-coughs and tumours of the face, and particularly of the eye-lids, were common to us in Dublin, and in the neighbouring counties of Kildare and Wicklow: one of theſe I met with was eryſipelatous, and accompanied with an acute fever.

The month of October was eminently diſtinguiſhed by the invaſion of an epidemic catarrhal fever. It had made its firſt appearance in London in Auguſt, and was at its heighth about the middle of

Sep-

September. It ſeems to have travelled gradually to the Weſt and North: for Briſtol and Cork had it in the beginning of October, whereas I did not hear of it in Dublin till the middle of that month. It viſited every province in this kingdom; the county of Weſtmeath had it later than we, and Lurgan in Ulſter, had it not till the fourteenth of November, when we were recovering*.

It attacked with ſhivering, ſoreneſs of the limbs, pains in the head and back, reſtleſſneſs, a cough and running at the noſe and eyes; and, in ſome, a delirium: ſome had ſore throats. Its firſt attack was mild, and the pulſe ſcarce advanced above the natural ſtroke; but in the progreſs of the diſeaſe, it was quicker, the urine redder, the blood ſizy, the pain of the head and limbs more ſevere. This deſcription agrees with Dr. Short's

* Short, on the Bills of Mortality, remarks, that moſt epidemic diſeaſes have their riſe in the South, and ſpread gradually to the North and Weſt of England.

account

account in his Chronological Hiſtory of the Weather and Seaſons, viz. that in Yorkſhire this catarrhous fever was more ſevere than that above in 1733, and that bleeding was more neceſſary.

By keeping confined and warm, it commonly vaniſhed in about three days: otherwiſe, it laſted much longer. Beſides the cough and running at the noſe and eyes, which in many were inflamed, ſweating was the diſcharge which relieved moſt, and on the firſt invaſion, on going to bed and drinking plentifully of thin diluting liquors, they fell almoſt inſtantly into profuſe ſweats, which took off their complaints in one day: ſo that it might be called an ephemera; but at the heighth it proved of four or five more days duration.

The aſthmatic and conſumptive were more vehemently affected by it, to many of whom in Dublin it proved mortal.

In London, at the heighth of this diſeaſe, their weekly bill roſe to near double

the

the uſual ſtandard, viz. to eight hundred and ſixty-one; but in Dublin, in the week ending October the twenty-eighth, the bill of mortality was increaſed to one hundred and forty-four, which was about three times the uſual number: whereas it will appear, that the reverſe of this obtained in the influenza, A. D. 1743 (the ſame diſeaſe under another name) viz. wherein in London their weekly bill roſe to treble, whereas in Dublin, it ſcarce roſe to double the uſual number; the reaſon of which difference it is very obvious to aſſign, viz. the difference of the ſeaſons in which theſe diſeaſes appeared in theſe places at theſe different times, viz. in the preſent year it arrived in Dublin further on in the winter than in London, where it arrived at its heighth in the middle of September; but it did not reach us till the middle of October: whereas in 1743, it appeared with us farther on in the ſpring, viz. in May, having viſited London in April, and conſequently with

us

us the warmth of the advancing ſeaſon promoted the natural criſis by the ſkin; whereas in the preſent year the daily advancing cold retarded it.

With this catarrhal fever were interſperſed ſome others of longer duration, but of a quite different nature; for this was a foreign diſeaſe ſui generis, which was neither prevented by the others, though attended alſo with a cough (ſeveral who had laboured under theſe being ſeized with this new infection in common with others) nor did it prevent coughs and peripneumonies in others, who were ſeized with theſe afterwards.

WINTER, 1737, 1738.

December. Moſtly cloudy, wet, windy, and foggy at intervals, but few fair days. The eighteenth a ſtorm at S. A little froſt with the fog, but not laſting. The principal wind S. W.

January. Cloudy, windy, and wet: for ſome time unuſually warm, and, contrary

to

to cuſtom, warmer than December. The ſixth, ſeventh, eighth, and ninth, ſtormy at S. W. The principal wind S. W.

February. Great variety and changes of weather, fair, cloudy, wet, windy; ſometimes warm like ſummer, then froſt, ſnow, and hail; and the twenty-ſeventh thunder and lightning. The principal winds S. W. N. W. S. and S. E.

SUMMARY.

Spring warm, and May exceſſively hot.

Summer moſtly fair, but great changes as to the temperature of the air; ſome days exceſſively hot, others very cold, and Auguſt a winter-like month.

Autumn fair and mild.

Winter open.

The months of December, January, and February, though in general very healthful, were not wholly exempt from fevers, ſome of which were of the low kind, and the pulſe ſcarce ſenſibly quick: one of theſe proved fatal on the fifth or ſixth day.

In

In February were violent colds, ſore throats, and ſome tumors of the parotids.

The ſum total of burials this year was two thouſand two hundred and ſeventeen.

SPRING.

March. The fore and greater part of the month alternately fair, cloudy, rainy, and ſometimes a little wind: it concluded with ſoft ſpring weather. Winds variable from N. W. S. W. and W. to N. E. N. and S.

April. The fore and greater part of the month alternately cloudy, ſhowery, and fair. From the nineteenth to the end a good deal of rain and cold weather, with hail. The winds S. E. W. N. W. N. E. and S. W.

May. Fair and cloudy weather interchangeably; and a good deal of rain. The principal wind S. E.

Agues, which had diſappeared ſince the two laſt hot ſummers, made their appearance again this ſpring, and even in June and

and July, and frequently diſguiſed under the appearance of other diſeaſes.

SUMMER.

June. A cold and wet month, but concluded hot. The principal winds S. W.

July. The prevailing weather was fair, and frequently hot, not without rain interſperſed. The twenty-eighth a ſtorm at W. N. W. The principal winds W. and S. W.

Auguſt. A wet and cold month generally. The principal winds W. and N. W.

The ſmall-pox was of a bad kind, and frequently mortal; but became very mild and favourable in Auguſt.

The month of June was not quite exempt from fevers, ſuch as deſcribed in the year 1736.

AUTUMN.

September. Generally wet and windy, and ſometimes cold to the ſeventeenth; the principal

principal wind S. W. The ninth a ſtorm at S. W. From the eighteenth to the end moſtly fair, and the wind N. E. S. E. and E.

October. A cloudy and rainy month, the winds W. N. W. S. E. S. and S. W.

November. Generally hazy and cloudy, with little rain to the nineteenth, and the wind S. E. with a high barometer: from the nineteenth to the end wet, and the wind S. W. The twentieth and twenty-fourth, ſtormy at S. W.

In the autumn, in ſeveral parts of the town, beſides violent colds and ſore throats, appeared alſo an acute fever of four, five, ſix, or ſeven days duration, attended with an inflammation in the throat and neighbouring glands, and an intenſe pain in the head. A large ſpontaneous ſweat proved critical to ſome of them: others had eruptions on the ſkin of various kinds.

WINTER, 1738, 1739.

December. The firſt ſeven days windy and wet. The ſixth and ſeventh ſtormy

at

at S. W. and N. W. with lightning; thence to the end of the month viciſſitudes of moiſt fogs, froſts, wind, and rain. The twenty-ſixth at night ſtormy at W. The principal winds W. and S. W.

January. Generally windy and wet. The thirteenth at night, and fourteenth in the morning, a ſultry day preceding, was a violent ſtorm at S. W. which was ſucceeded by good weather for five days following. The principal winds W. and S. W.

February. The four firſt days moſtly fair, thence to the fourteenth generally windy or wet: the eleventh and twelfth, a ſtorm at S. W. which, as that of the foregoing month, was preceded by ſultry weather. The principal winds W. and S. W.

SUMMARY.

Spring ſeaſonable.

Summer cold and wet, except July, which was hot and dry.

Autumn

Autumn for the moſt part wet.

Winter wet and ſtormy.

The months of December, January, and February, though very wet and windy, were remarkably healthful.

The ſum total of burials this year was two thouſand five hundred and ſix.

SPRING, 1739.

March. Moſtly fair the firſt ſeven days, otherwiſe unuſually cold and froſty, and much more remarkable for froſt, hail, and ſnow, than wind; particularly from the tenth, to the twenty-firſt, with N. and N. E. winds. It concluded hazy and cloudy, with W. and S. W. winds.

April. Alternately fair and ſhowery as uſual; but the general temperature of the month was unuſually cold, with frequent ſnow and hail, to the great prejudice of the vegetables. The principal winds the fore part of the month, N. and N. W. the latter N. E, and S. E.

May.

May. The preceding half of the month alternately fair, cloudy, and wet, and the principal winds S. E. The other half was fair. The twenty-ſecond thunder and ſhowers, and the principal winds E. and N. E.

The ſpring, eſpecially March and April, were attended with colds, a few eruptive fevers, and ſome intermitting ones. In May appeared divers inflammatory diſorders affecting the jaws, face, and eyes, and ſome miliary fevers, both which alſo attended the month of June.

SUMMER.

June. Excepting a very few hot and fair days with S. E. and E. winds, the month was generally moiſt and cold, and the principal winds W. and S. W.

July. Unuſually cold and moiſt, the thermometer not higher than in May; but the hygrometer was heavier than in the two laſt months. Few days without rain, except from the fifteenth to the twenty-

twenty-ſecond. The principal winds to the eleventh S. W. thence to the end N. N. E. or N. W.

Auguſt. The firſt nine days variable, and the winds N. N. W. E. and S. E. From the ninth to the twentieth fair, and the winds E. and S. E. thence to the end rainy, and moſtly S. W. and it concluded N. W. and cold, wet and windy.

The latter part of July, and the months of Auguſt, September, and October, were infeſted with a fever, which was very frequent during this period, not unlike that of the autumn of the preceding year; with which compare alſo the years 1741, 1745, 1748. It was attended with an intenſe pain in the head. It terminated ſometimes in four, for the moſt part in five or ſix days, ſometimes in nine, and commonly in a critical ſweat: it was far from being mortal. I was aſſured of ſeventy of the poorer ſort at the ſame time in this fever, abandoned to the uſe of whey and God's good providence, who all

all recovered. The crisis, however, was very imperfect, for they were subject to relapses, even sometimes to the third time; nor did their urine come to a complete separation.

Divers of them, as their fever declined, had a paroxysm in the evening, and in some there succeeded pains in the limbs.

AUTUMN.

September. Generally very wet: the tenth at night a great storm of rain and wind at N. some interpositions of fair weather: the winds variable, S. W. S. W. N. W. S. E. E. N. and N. E.

October. Generally dry and foggy to the twenty-fifth, and sometimes cold, and the winds S. E. and N. E. thence to the end wet and stormy, S. W. and N. W. and concluded windy at S. E.

November. Alternities of rain, frost, stormy and mostly foggy weather, and the winds accordingly variable from E. to S. E. W. S. and N. W.

In

In October appeared ſome dyſenteries; and in October, November, and December, beſides cold, we had anomalous meaſles, eryſipelas's and inflammations about the neck and face.

WINTER, 1739, 1740.

December for the moſt part fair, but with moiſt fogs and froſt interpoſed: from the fifth to the ninth, wet and windy at S. W. which was the prevailing wind the fore part of the month. From the twenty-ſeventh to the end a moſt intenſe froſt, and attended with a high wind intolerably piercing at S. E. and E.

January. The froſt concluding the laſt month continued throughout this: the greateſt intenſity of cold was at the twenty-ſeventh at night; the month concluded with a S. E. wind, attended with a gradual, but not durable thaw.

February. The froſt continued, though with a little interruption to the fourteenth; with winds S. E. and N. E. then ſucceeded a coma complete thaw, with alternities of clouds, rain, and fair weather: winds N. W. W. and S. W.

SUMMARY.

Spring moſtly cold.

Summer very wet.

Autumn variable.

Winter froſty, after a long ſeries of open winters.

December was not free from other inflammatory diſorders, beſides thoſe mentioned laſt autumn, which grew more violent the two following months of January and February, the time of the great froſt, which was very prolific in coughs, attended with ſore throats, pleuriſies, and peripneumonies, which were very frequent both in the town and country. They bore bleeding well, and the blood was ſizy; and no wonder intenſe cold producing the ſame effects as intenſe heat, viz. a denſity of the blood, and a conſtriction of the veſſels.

It

It was a fatal ſeaſon to many, not only the old, infirm, and aſthmatic, but to children alſo. Our weekly bill roſe in theſe two months to one hundred and thirty and one hundred and forty, near triple the ordinary number.

It was worthy of obſervation, as an inſtance of the effects of viciſſitudes in the weather, that many ſickened on the thaw who had been well in the froſt, which Wintringham alſo obſerves to have happened in the inflammatory diſeaſes attendant on ſuch ſeaſons*: and from hence we may learn the neceſſity of a retroſpection, as well as a preſent view of the ſtate of the weather, which may be further illuſtrated by another obſervation, viz. that divers diſeaſes which appear in autumn, do rage more violently according to the degree of the heat of the preceding ſummer, which heat laid the foundation for

* The ſprings of watches, which are apt to be affected by ſevere froſts, do not commonly break till the thaw.

thoſe

thofe diforders raging more on the fucceeding ftoppage of perfpiration in autumn.

The fum total of burials this year was two thoufand two hundred and one.

SPRING, 1740.

March. There was a little mild weather at the beginning, but it was generally a very dry and dufty March, and the principal winds were at fome point of the N.

April. A preternaturally cold and dry month, little falling weather but hail or fnow. The principal winds E. and N. E. The fpring fix weeks more backward than ufual.

May. Froft and fnow at the beginning: the difpofition to drought continued, though there were fome rainy days. The principal wind N. E.

In the fpring pleurifies, peripneumonies, quinfies, tumours of the parotids, and ophthalmies were frequent.

The fmall pox began to rage in May, of which more in fummer.

SUM-

SUMMER.

June dry, and from the ſeventeenth to the twenty-fourth hot, and the principal winds at ſome point of the N. or E.

July. The weather was variable; yet ſtill the N. winds prevailed; and there was ſome froſt and ice this month.

Auguſt. Generally moiſt: the ſixth a ſtorm at S. W. The winds variable, S. E. W. S. W. and S. for the moſt part.

The ſmall-pox, which began to rage in May, increaſed with the ſummer; ſo that in July ſixteen died of that diſeaſe in a week (a far greater number than uſual) and in Auguſt twenty-two and thirty-three. At the ſame time they were ſtill much more mortal at Cork than here; and were alſo mortal at London and at Plymouth at the ſame time.

Dyſenteries made their appearance in July, as they did alſo at the ſame time at Plymouth, of which more in autumn and winter.

A U-

AUTUMN.

September. Through the greater half of the month were frequent rains and ſometimes winds, generally at S. W. thence to the end ſerene; it concluded froſty, and the winds at ſome point of the E. or N.

October. Frequent froſts throughout the month, and the principal winds from ſome point of the N. or E. The thirty-firſt a ſtorm.

November. Froſts frequent, and much more than of late years, and the principal winds N. and N. W. Some winds, particularly a ſtorm the twenty-firſt at night at S. W. with thunder and lightning.

The dyſenteries, which began in July, continued through the autumn and winter; having firſt begun among the poor (ſeveral of whom died for want) they ſpread to the rich.

N. B. There was a great dearth of proviſions this autumn, which proceeded

almoſt

almoſt to a famine in winter; the potatoes having failed, whilſt other proviſions bore double or treble their uſual price.

In autumn alſo appeared an epidemic continual fever, which did not wholly ceaſe in winter; of which in the following year.

WINTER, 1740, 1741.

December. Variable at the beginning and end of the month: from the eighth to the twenty-firſt froſty. The twenty-firſt the thaw was followed by a violent ſtorm at S. E. The principal winds from ſome point of the N. or E.

January. Hazy, wet, and windy at times: froſt from the ſixth to the ſixteenth. Winds E. and S. E.

February. The foregoing half of the month variable, with interpoſitions of rain and wind, which was generally at S. W. The ſixteenth a ſtorm at S. W. From the ſixteenth to the twenty-fourth froſty, and the winds at N. E. and E.

SUM-

SUMMARY.

Spring dry and cold.

Summer dry, with a predominance of northerly winds.

Autumn unuſually froſty, with a continued prevalence of N. and E. winds.

Winter froſty, with a continued prevalence of N. and E. winds.

The ſum total of burials this year was three thouſand three hundred and four.

SPRING, 1741.

March. Serene, dry, froſty, and duſty, and the winds E. S. E. and N. E. blaſting and burning the graſs, ſo that we had leſs ſpring by far than in February.

April. Unuſually dry: ſhowers exceedingly rare: duſty, like a ſummer month; and the N. and E. winds ſtill prevailed.

May. The great drought of the two preceding months continued throughout the greateſt part of this, and the general courſe of the winds was E. S. E. N. E. and

and N. From the eleventh to the ſix-teenth very cold.

Beſides colds and inflammatory diſorders as laſt ſpring, and famine among ſome of the poor, the dyſentery raged greatly, particularly in March, when in Dublin that article amounted to twenty-one in a week, when it arrived at its greateſt heighth, though it was leſs mortal than in the country, to which the better care taken of the poor, and of their food, undoubtedly contributed.

The fever which had begun laſt autumn returned in ſpring, of which more in the ſequel.

In this morbid conſtitution ſucceeding the great froſt in 1739, we have a ſtrong confirmation of the truth of Wintringham's obſervation of the unwholeſomeneſs of a long continued drought, and E. winds in theſe iſlands.

SUMMER.

June. The long and ſevere drought was now tempered by frequent ſhowers: the

the nineteenth thunder-ſhowers: the twentieth and twenty-firſt ſtormy at S. W. The fourteenth, and from the twenty-fourth to the end ſerene and hot, the winds variable.

July. The preceding half of the month generally ſerene, and the wind moſtly N. E. The latter half of the month frequent ſhowers, and the wind moſtly S. W. Several very hot days, particularly the ninth, tenth, twenty-fifth, and twenty-ſixth.

Auguſt. Generally hot and dry, and more hot days than in the laſt month. Wind N. W.

The fever, which had begun laſt autumn, returned in ſpring, and raged through the ſummer. It was common to this city, to Cork, Briſtol, and London, and often eluded the ſkill of phyſicians. It raged through the provinces of Munſter, Leinſter, and Ulſter; but was moſt fatal to the firſt, where their poor were worſe provided for, from whom the diſeaſe ſpread to the richer ſort; and it was computed that one fifth part of the inhabitants died,

though

though probably with exaggeration. The mortality increafed with the advancing feafon; and with us, in Dublin, arrived at its heighth about the end of Auguft; for on the twenty-eighth of that month the article of fevers in our weekly bills, amounted to thirty, above double their late ufual number.

For a minute defcription of this fever, I refer to Dr. Connell's Obfervationes Medicinales: it fhall fuffice for me to point out fome of its moft diftinguifhing attendants, viz.

The firft attack was commonly very mild and deceitful; fo that at the beginning it was frequently fuppofed to be no more than a common cold: whence a neglect of early confinement, and a proper regimen, was often attended by fatal confequences.

The pulfe, though variable in different fubjects, and at different times of the difeafe, I obferved feveral times to be fcarce quicker than in health, even on the fixth, feventh, and eighth days.

The

The ſpots which ſometimes attended (though not eſſentially) were moſtly of a duſky red, ſometimes purple, and ſometimes intermixed with miliary puſtules; and Dr. Connell in Munſter obſerved, that, profuſe hemorrhages at the noſe moſt uſually attended; but theſe were not ſo frequent with us, the diſeaſe here being leſs violent and leſs fatal; nor was the blood always in a colliquative ſtate, but ſometimes ſizy, as the above named author alſo remarks*.

A delirium, coma, and ſpaſms, commonly cloſed the tragical ſcene, in which bliſters had very little ſucceſs, even when applied after bleeding and other evacuations; and as many miſcarried under the uſe of bliſters, ſo they did under that of the moſt generous cordials and great plenty of ſack, which had no effect in

* So Huxham obſerves a ſizy blood to be frequent in the beginning of malignant fevers; and yet that blood drawn two or three days after from the ſame perſon, hath been quite looſe, diſſolved, and as it were ſanious.

raiſing

raiſing the depreſſed pulſe: on the other hand, it was obſerved, that many of the poor, abandoned through neceſſity to a low aceſcent diet, and ſome of them drinking nothing but water, recovered.

This may afford a profitable hint in practice, with regard to ſuch fevers as theſe, being of the putrid kind; even as in the bilious fever of Barbadoes, which is alſo of this kind, in which the coma, tremors, and ſubſultus have been obſerved to be increaſed by bliſters, and the hemorrhages likewiſe to be haſtened or increaſed by them *.

Another notable circumſtance ſeems worthy of being recorded, in relation to the ſubjects which this fever generally attacked, both here and in England, viz. that they were generally men, and thoſe of a middle age, and ſtrong, and but few women; alſo children were more rarely attacked †.

* Hilary of the Weather and Diſeaſes of Barbadoes.

† Theſe different effects of the predominant, exceſſive, and unuſual drought which egregiouſly obtained previous

It ſeems alſo not unworthy of notice, that through the three ſummer months, there was frequent here and there a fever altogether, without the malignity attending the former, of ſix or ſeven days duration, terminating in a critical ſweat, as did the other alſo frequently; but in this the patients were ſubject to a relapſe, even to a third or fourth time, and yet recovered.

previous to and during the preſent morbid conſtitution on the bodies of men, and thoſe of women and children reſpectively, are perfectly agreeable to ancient obſervation, as appears from the following paſſage in Celſus: "Si ſicca æſtas aquilones habuit, & autumnus quoque ſiccus iiſdem quoque aquilonibus perflatur, omnibus quidem mollioribus corporibus, inter quæ muliebria, ſecunda valetudo contingit, durioribus vero inſtare poſſunt & aridæ lippitudines, & febres, partim acutæ, partim longæ, & hi morbi, qui ex atra bile naſcuntur."

And it may be worth obſerving, that, in the fever which raged on that called the black aſſizes at Oxford, though it ſpared no complexion nor conſtitution, yet, it chiefly attacked the bilious; nor did any woman or child die of it, and the poor were exempt from it. PHILOS. TRANS. Vol. L. Part II.

A U-

AUTUMN.

September. Great varieties of weather with reſpect to heat and cold, dryneſs and moiſture. The ſeventh at night a great ſtorm at E. The winds alſo were extremely variable.

October. The winds and weather variable as the laſt month. The eighteenth, nineteenth, and twentieth, ſtormy at S. W.

November. The winds and weather variable: ſome froſts.

The malignant fever, of which above, as alſo the dyſentery, though abated in autumn, did not entirely ceaſe.

It was computed that eighty thouſand died in this kingdom of the fever, dyſentery, and famine, in the years 1740, 1741 *.

WINTER, 1741, 1742.

December. Generally foggy and froſty, with ſome rain interſperſed. The principal winds E. S. E. and N. E.

* Connell Obſervationes Medicinales.

Janu-

January. The firſt twelve days variable, viz. windy, wet, ſerene, and ſometimes froſty, and the winds variable. From the thirteenth to the end of the month ſtormy at S. W.

February. The ſtormy weather of laſt month, continued the firſt ſeven days of this, and was ſucceeded by variable weather to the fifteenth; and the winds hitherto W. and S. W. from thence to the end froſt and ſnow, and the wind S. W. then N. S. E. and E.

SUMMARY.

Spring exceſſively dry, with a continuance of E. and N. winds.

Summer hot, much more than of late.

Autumn variable in winds and weather.

A ſecond froſty winter, with an interpoſition of variable and ſtormy weather.

The winter concluded healthy, and the bills of mortality ſunk conſpicuouſly on the ſtormy weather: and Short remarks, that the high winds in January put an entire ſtop to the fever in Yorkſhire.

The

The ſum total of burials this year was two thouſand ſeven hundred and ninety-two.

N. B. This morbid conſtitution ſeems to bear a conſiderable analogy to that obſerved by Sydenham, in the year 1665, after a very cold winter and dry ſpring; which was alſo attended with pleuriſies, peripneumonies, quinſies, and other inflammatory diſorders, which proved very mortal, and withal a peſtilential fever, and then the peſtilence itſelf.

And perhaps the following anecdote from Dr. Berkley, biſhop of Cloyne, conſiſting of facts wherein there could hardly be a miſtake, may deſerve attention, viz.

" In the ſickly ſeaſon 1741, were twenty five fevers in the biſhop's own family, which were cured by tar-water drank copiouſly; and the ſame method was practiſed by ſeveral of his poor neighbours with equal ſucceſs. It ſuddenly calmed the feveriſh anxieties; and it was found that without bleeding, vomiting,

bliſtering,

bliftering, or any other evacuation or medicine, very bad fevers could be cured, viz. by the fole drinking of tar-water milk-warm, and in good quantity, as a large glafs every hour in bed: and it was obfervable, that fuch as were cured by this comfortable cordial, recovered health and fpirits at once; while thofe who had been cured by evacuations, languifhed long before they recovered."

SPRING, 1742.

March. Extremely dufty, fcarce any rain or high winds: generally ferene and cold: the winds N.E. N.W. S.E. and E.

April. The drought of laft month continued through this, which was deftitute of its ufual fhowers, except of hail at the beginning: the winds N.W. N. N.E. W. E. and S.E*.

* The end of April was exceffively hot and dry, like the middle of fummer, fo that the flies appeared.

May.

May. The drought of laſt month continued to the ſixth of this: thence to the thirteenth, ſerene and cold, and the winds N. N.E. and N.W. thence to the end rain and fair weather interchangeably, and the winds W. S.W. S.E. and E.

The cold and dry ſpring was attended with diſorders not unlike thoſe of the two preceding dry and cold ſprings, particularly colds and chin-coughs; and the meaſles were exceedingly frequent. The infirm, both young and old, and particularly the aſthmatic, ſuffered greatly, and not leſs remarkably than did the vegetables, during this ſharp cold ſeaſon and prevalence of the N.E. winds; and the colds affected not only mankind, but the horſes; and was fatal to ſeveral, both here and in England, particularly at Plymouth, where Huxham obſerves, that in March almoſt all the horſes out of the ſtable had the mange and a purulent cough.

SUMMER.

June. The firſt half of the month moſtly ſerene, and the winds variable; yet gene-

generally at ſome point of the E. the latter half frequent ſhowers, often ſultry, and ſometimes a little thunder. The winds S. E. S. and S. W.

July. Frequent ſhowers were interſperſed through the greateſt part of the month, and it was cool: the winds variable, but concluded hot; the wind E.

Auguſt. Serene and warm weather: a long continued ſummer: the winds E. and S. E.

The ſummer was more healthful than the ſpring, and the fever mentioned laſt year was far leſs frequent, and diſappeared entirely in winter.

AUTUMN.

September. Variable as to ſerenity, wind, heat, and cold; the winds variable.

October. Generally very windy and wet. The ſecond, tenth, and eleventh, ſtormy at S. W. The winds generally between S. and W. there were alſo frequent ſlight froſts.

No-

November. The beginning ſtormy and the wind W. thence to the end interpoſitions of hail, ſnow, and froſt, and frequent fogs; and the principal winds W. N. E. E. and S. E.

The autumn produced but few diſeaſes.

WINTER, 1742, 1743.

December. The firſt half of the month generally froſty, and the wind S. E. the remaining part of the month frequent ſtorms, and wind at S. W.

January. The ſtormy weather of laſt month continued with rain the firſt ſeven days of this, and the wind W. and S. W. thence to the twenty-ſecond alternities of fog, froſt, cloudy weather, and rain, and the winds E. S. E. W. and S. W. thence to the end very ſtormy, and the wind S. W.

February. The wet and windy weather of laſt month continued the firſt fourteen days of this, and the winds generally between S. and W. The third a great ſtorm at S. and S. S. E. From the fourteenth to the twentieth ſerene, the

winds

winds as before: thence to the end wet and windy, the winds W. S. W. and N. W.

SUMMARY.

Spring exceſſively dry, as the two laſt years, with a continued prevalence of N. and E. winds.

A ſecond hot ſummer.

The autumn variable.

Winter ſtormy, yet not without conſiderable froſts interpoſed.

Proviſions, this winter, were as plentiful as they had been ſcarce for the two laſt years: bread was ſold at twenty-one pounds ſix ounces for a ſhilling, and the winter quarter was remarkably healthy and ſtormy.

The ſum total of burials this year was two thouſand three hundred and twenty.

SPRING, 1743.

March. A very cold month, frequent froſts, ſnow, and hail. The winds variable.

April.

April. The frofty weather of laft month continued the firft feven days of this, with hail and fnow, and N. and N. W. winds: the reft of the month feafonable interpofitions of fhowers as ufual, and the winds S. W. S. E. E. and N. E.

May. Warm and unufually dry weather for the firft thirteen days, and the winds E. fucceeded by a fudden coldnefs of fome days, and the winds more N. thence to the end wet and windy at times, and the winds W. and S. W.

The fpring was not exempt from colds and inflammatory diforders, quinzies, ophthalmies, &c. But in April the influenza or catarrh, which had made its firft appearance at Rome (where it fwept away multitudes, as it did afterwards in Spain) reached London, where it proved fatal to feveral, efpecially the old and infirm; and advanced their weekly bills to one thoufand one hundred, and one thoufand five hundred, near treble the ufual number: but it did not arrive in Dublin until May,

where

where it was milder and lefs fatal than in London, our weekly bill at its greateft height, May twenty, being only fixty-feven, which falls greatly fhort of the above proportion of deaths in London; as alfo far fhort of the number dying in the two refembling epidemic diforders of 1732, 1733, and 1737, defcribeda bove, the firft of which was at the latter end of winter and beginning of fpring, the latter in October: whereas this made its attack on us here at the end of the fpring, a feafon lefs favourable to the difeafe, as more encouraging the neceffary perfpiration, by which the diftemper was ufually carried off. Compare alfo the year 1762, where is a return of the like epidemic.

It vifited the remote parts of Ulfter and Munfter, fcarce fparing a family, and fpread itfelf over Europe like the two epidemic diforders above mentioned.

Foreftus mentions an epidemical cough and catarrh, which over ran all Europe in fix weeks time, of which fcarce one in a thou-

thousand died; from which however the influenza differed, proving fatal to several.

The attack was like that of a violent cold tending to a fever, it being truly a catarrhal fever. It began commonly with horrors, a great pain in the head and back, soreness of the chest and limbs, in some sore throats, lowness of spirits attended in others, and in some a slight delirium, in others a vomiting attended.

The tongue was for the most part white, the pulse but rarely quick, the blood sizy.

The natural crisis was by sweat, the first or second day, though in some weakly persons the sweat was protracted till the third or fourth day, and some held out to the fourteenth and twenty-first day, and died.

It was observed to leave the hypochondriacal weak and low for a considerable time. It proved fatal to many of the old, infirm, asthmatic, and tabid.

I ob-

I obſerved ſome remains of it to continue with us to the latter end of July.

Now in order to illuſtrate the above hiſtory, and to take off ſurprize from the leſs learned reader, I ſhall here exhibit, from the collections of the indefatigable Dr. Short, in his Chronological Hiſtory of the Weather and Seaſons, an account of ſome other notable epidemics in ſeveral reſpects ſimilar to this, viz.

1. The Sudor Anglicus, which made its fiſt appearance in England in the year 1485, when it was very fatal, killing many in three or four hours, and in ſome towns a half, in others a third, of their inhabitants.

Its ſecond viſit was in 1506, when it was not ſo fatal as before, the remedy being found out, viz. going to bed, and promoting large ſweats for a day.

It differed remarkably from the influenza in the ſubjects it attacked, which were moſtly ſtrong perſons between thirty and

and fifty, and rarely affected the old, which the influenza attacked moſt.

2. In the year 1688, in the middle of May, a fever began, at London, which ſpread over all England, and likewiſe over all Ireland in July: alſo it ſpread over all Europe from eaſt to weſt. It ſeldom held the ſick above two or three days, except they were let blood, and then it laſted ſeven or eight before the ſweat (which was the general criſis) began.

Not one of fifteen eſcaped, yet not one of a thouſand died; and it was obſerved both in England and Ireland ſome time before the fever began, that a ſlight, but univerſal diſeaſe, ſeized the horſes, viz. a great defluction of rheum from their noſes.

3. A like diſorder prevailed alſo A. D. 1691, in many parts of Europe, in London, and afterwards in Dublin, travelling from eaſt to weſt, as did the influenza, and likewiſe the catarrhal fever of 1732, and 1737.

4. The

4. The Dunkirk fever, ſo called from its being brought by ſoldiers from that place, which appeared in London in 1713, * having probably had its original from the plague which broke out a few years before at Dantzick, began only with a pain in the head, and went off uſually in large ſweats after a day's confinement; but at Dunkirk it was attended with the additional ſymptoms of vomiting, diarrhœa, &c..

Dr. Short adds to the ſymptoms a ſevere dry cough, and ſays that ſweating and diuretics were the cure, but bleeding was very pernicious or fatal.

5. The diſeaſe called coccaluche or coccalucio (becauſe the ſick wore a cap or covering cloſe all over their heads) came from the iſland Melite in Africa into Sicily, A. D. 1510, ſo into Spain and Italy, and thence over the Alps into Portugal, Hungary, and a great part of Germany, even to the Baltic Sea, every month ſhift-

* Mead on the Plague.

ing

ing its ſituation with the wind, ſo into France, Britain, &c. raging over all Europe, not miſſing a family, ſcarce a perſon. This alſo was an epidemic catarrh, and was attended with a grievous pain in the head, hoarſeneſs, difficulty of breathing, and a teazing cough, threatening ſuffocation. The firſt days it was without ſpitting; but the ſeventh or eighth day much phlegm was ſpit up, and then the cough and ſhortneſs of breath were eaſier. None died except ſome children. In ſome it went off with a looſeneſs, in others by ſweating; bleeding and purging did hurt *.

This diſorder appeared again A. D. 1557, 1580, and 1597. So far Dr. Short.

SUMMER.

June. Generally ſerene and dry, though from the twelfth to the eighteenth remarkably cold: the month concluded warm. The winds variable.

* Short's Chronological hiſtory of the Weather and Diſeaſes.

July.

July. Frequent ſhowers throughout the month, and ſometimes ſultry. The winds variable.

Auguſt. Generally ſerene and hot, and the principal winds at ſome point of the E. The thermometer higher than for ſome years paſt.

AUTUMN.

September. The weather was very variable, the beginning generally cold, and the winds W. and N. W. The middle of the month warm and ſummer-like, and the winds S. E. The end cold and the winds N. E. S. E. and N. W.

October. Generally ſerene and dry the foregoing half of the month: the latter half frequent rains and ſome little froſt, and ſometimes ſultry, and concluded ſtormy. The winds variable.

November. The windy and wet weather continued the firſt ſix days, the winds W. and S. W. This was ſucceeded by froſt and N. and N. W. winds;

and

and this by dark mizzling weather, the winds N. E. S. E. S. W. and S. The month concluded warm and ſummer-like, with S. W. and S. winds.

The ſummer and autumn were remarkable for health, as well as for fertility and plenty in large crops of corn of all ſorts; and we had ſcarce any diſeaſes then or in winter, except colds and ſore throats, from which we are ſeldom long exempted.

Throughout the hot month of Auguſt were frequent, both among children and adults, white tubercles on the ſkin, as from the ſtinging of nettles (the eſſere Arabum) but no way dangerous, nor requiring the aſſiſtance of the phyſician.

WINTER, 1743, 1744.

December. Generally froſty and foggy, and the principal winds S. E. N. W. W. and E.

January the prevailing weather of the

the month was frosty, and the winds variable.

February. Mostly fair the first half of the month, and the winds variable: the latter half of the month wet and windy, the winds S. W. and S. W. The eighteenth at night a great storm at W. and again the twenty-eighth at S. W.

SUMMARY.

Spring variable, less unseasonable than the springs of the three last years, though still inclined to cold.

Summer mostly serene, hot, and dry.

Autum variable.

Winter frosty, and concluded stormy.

Besides the sore throats endemial to this country, there raged this autumn and winter (having begun in summer, and which was not extinct for many years after) an epidemic disease, which might pass under * that general denomination, but was of a

* It also began in France in the year 1743, and returned at different times after.

species

ſpecies wholly diſtinct, being very malignant and fatal to children, and eluding the ſkill of phyſicians.

It raged in ſome of the neighbouring as well as remote counties, particularly in the county of Wicklow, Carlow, Queen's County, Kilkenny, Cavan, Roſcommon, Leitrem, Sligo, and perhaps many others, carrying off incredible numbers, and ſometimes ſweeping away the children of whole villages in a few days: however, there were but very few inſtances of it in Dublin, the ſmoak of the city perhaps correcting the morbid effluvia, as in divers other epidemics; and therefore phyſicians in the country were beſt able to give a deſcription of this diſeaſe, and of the methods purſued for the cure of it, who, however, as far as I have learnt, have been profoundly ſilent on this ſubject, although ſo deeply intereſting, and the diſeaſe ſo deſtructive and reproachful to their art; nor is it to be doubted but accounts of ſuch diſorders communicated

to

to the public, and compared, together with the various endeavours ufed to cure them, might have ftarted very ufeful hints.

It is probable that we had this diforder here, as early as we have any accounts of the malignant fore throat in England, which though not in all refpects like ours, yet the moft probable method of cure feems in both to be the fame, which method a correfpondent of mine in the country, Doctor Molloy, had the fagacity to ftrike out long before any accounts of their malignant fore throat in England were publifhed, which, together with his defcription of the difeafe, I fhall here infert, viz.

" It is peculiar to children, and thofe chiefly of from a month to three, four, five, fix, eight, or nine years old. They commonly, for a day or wo, or more, had a little hoarfenefs, fometimes a little cough; then in an inftant they were feized with a great fuffocation, lafting a minute or two, and their face became livid:

livid: they have frequent returns of theſe fits of ſuffocation like aſthmatic perſons. The ſaid ſuffocation is ever followed by one ſymptom, which continues till they die, viz. a prodigious rattling in the upper part of the aſpera arteria, reſembling that ſound which attends colds where there is phlegm that cannot be got up. It is ſcarcē ſenſible when they are awake, but very great when they are aſleep."

The chief ſeat of the diſeaſe ſeems to be in the glottis, not far in the aſpera arteria. They have no difficulty of ſwallowing, nor does there appear the leaſt ſwelling inwardly or outwardly, though the uvula and parts about it are intenſely red.

Every one that is able, at ſome time or other of the diſeaſe, but generally at the beginning, throws up, by a ſlight cough, ſome florid, dilute blood. They have for the moſt part a diſpoſition to vomit, which when they do, they throw up a vaſt quantity of extremely viſcid matter.

They

They have no thirſt, nor do I perceive any quickneſs in their pulſe *: alſo their urine and ſtools are in a natural way. They have generally a clammy ſweat on them, and their breath is fetid.

Their death is generally ſudden, and when leaſt expected, the pulſe being good a minute before. Many die in twenty-four hours, none live above five days. Some have tumours behind the ears, which mortify: many have a prodigious weeping behind the ears, which is very corroſive.

I have tried evacuations of all kinds: frequent bleeding and ſevere bliſtering were of no ſervice.

A certain child recovered by a very profuſe ſweat, which came naturally, and continued two days and nights; this put me upon the following experiments: I ordered that the children who took this diſ-

* So Short in his Chronological Hiſtory of the Weather and Seaſons obſerves, in the malignant ſore throat at its firſt appearance in England, A. D. 1742, the pulſe and urine to be as in health: but in 1744, 45, 46, it was attended with a putrid fever and petechiæ.

order

order ſhould be firſt put into the warm bath, and that a ſweat ſhould be forced by ſack-whey, or a bolus of theriaca andromachi and camphor. Thoſe who ſweated by this means recovered, but thoſe that did not ſweat, died. So far my correſpondent.

Tournefort, in his Voyage to the Levant, mentions a diſeaſe, which ſeems to have borne a conſiderable reſemblance to this; and the method of cure may ſerve as an illuſtration and confirmation of that above propoſed, viz. it is frequent in the Levant, and peculiar to infants, whom it kills in forty-eight hours, being truly a carbuncle in the bottom of the throat, accompanied with a fever. The beſt method is to vomit inſtantly upon the firſt ſeizure, and to repeat the vomit, and keep up the ſtrength by cordials, particularly by theriaca, ſal volatile, and the like; and the ſolution of liquid ſtorax is an excellent gargle in this caſe.

In the year 1748, Dr. Fothergill publiſhed

liſhed an accurate account of the ſore throat attended with ulcers, which had appeared of late years in London, and the parts adjacent, which, among other appellations, is diſtinguiſhed by thoſe of angina maligna, and carbunculus anginoſus, which, with reſpect to the ſubjects it attacked, the tendency of the parts to mortification, and the method of cure alſo, bore a great reſemblance to ours; altho' it muſt be owned that the ſeat of the diſeaſe was different, being in ours chiefly the organs of reſpiration, in the other thoſe of deglutition, with a tumor in the uvula and tonſils, not obſervable in ours; as alſo a quickneſs of pulſe in that, which, according to my correſpondent above, did not attend ours.

But what agrees more exactly to ours is the charactereſtic ſymptom I find deſcribed in number four hundred and ninety-five of the Philoſophical Tranſactions, by Dr. Starr, under the name of morbus ſtrangulatorius, thus:

"An

" An occult angina, or morbus ſtrangulatorius, has within theſe four years (viz. preceding the year 1749) reigned in ſeveral parts of Cornwall with great ſeverity, and ſwept away whole families of children.

" In all theſe are ſigns of a putrid diſpoſition in the juices, v. g. in ſome corroſive ulcers in the groin, and about the anus, eating deep and threatening mortification; but the pathognomonic ſigns are a ſhort, low, hecking cough, productive of a difficult, noiſy, and ſtrangulating reſpiration.

" The matter ſpit up was very like jelly, mixed with a white opaque thready matter, ſomewhat reſembling a rotten membranous bag or ſlough, and it is truly in part membranous, conſiſting of the mucous coat of the larynx and aſpera arteria, with a viſcid matter ſticking to it like bird-lime;" and he concludes with this mournful obſervation, "that no remedy has yet been found for it;" from whence the

ſupe-

ſuperior malignity of this diſeaſe, as well as of ours above deſcribed, appears: for in 1748, when Dr. Fothergill publiſhed his account of the angina above mentioned in and about London, he ſays it was ſo mild as ſeldom to prove fatal, unleſs ill treated, or meeting with a bad ſubject, the morbid miaſmata having been perhaps partly weakened by time, and partly corrected by the effluvia of the city: however, the method propoſed in ours above agrees very nearly to what has been found moſt ſucceſsful in the other; bleeding, purging, and antiphlogiſtic medicines (the proper remedy in the common angina) having been found of no ſervice at all, but rather prejudicial: but, on the contrary, the warm cordial and alexipharmic regimen and medicines, have been attended with encouraging ſucceſs, which is agreeable to the obſervation of Huxham on the malignant ulcerous ſore throat which raged at Plymouth from the year 1751 to 1753, that whenever moderate, equally diffuſed ſweats

came

came on the third, fourth, or fifth day, or later, they were critical and ſalutary.

Dr. Short ſent me the following account of the further progreſs and different appearances put on by this diſeaſe, viz.

"It never left Sheffield entirely ſince the year 1745. Sometimes it was much milder; but in July 1759, it returned again in a violent, epidemic, contagious, and fatal manner, and, beſides others, cut off whole families of children. Now the ſymptoms were different from thoſe in 1741, for a briſk fever attended, which was followed by great ſickneſs and pukings, which continued ſome hours, and when theſe abated, a diarrhœa ſucceeded, and the greater the diarrhœa, the more violent the ſymptoms: the next day the tonſils began to ſwell, as alſo the face, which ſeemed œdematous, then eruptions like the meaſles broke out all over the body: about two days after, a ſanious humour began

to

to flow from the noſtrils, and often from the eyes. The ſwelling in the face kept increaſing, and the tonſils grew much larger, till about the ninth or eleventh day, when the ſick died as it were ſuffocated by the deluge of phlegm which had fallen upon the tonſils, uvula, and larynx; none had a peripneumony.

" In ſome there was an efflore ſcence on the ſkin like the ſcarlet fever, and theſe recovered.

" All evacuations and antiphlogiſtics were fatal; warming attenuant medicines ſucceeded beſt."

Rotheram, March 26, 1760.

For further ſatisfaction on this ſubject, I refer to Dr. Home's Enquiry into the Nature, Cauſe, and Cure, of the Croup, publiſhed at Edinburgh 1765, a diſeaſe which agrees well to that above deſcribed by my Iriſh correſpondent, and to the abovementioned morbus ſtrangulatorius of Dr. Starr, in the moſt eſſential and diſtintinguiſhing ſymptoms and circumſtances, viz. in the noiſe and ſuffocation in breathing; in its ſudden and ſurpriſing fatality; in the membranous-like bag, which is ſometimes ſpitted up; in the ſeat of the diſeaſe; and in the ſubjects it attacked.

The ſum total of burials this year was two thouſand one hundred and ninety-three.

SPRING, 1744.

March. Generally windy, with great rains, ſnow and hail, and the principal winds at ſome point of the N. or E.

N. B. There has been more rain ſince the middle of February laſt, than ſince the great froſt in 1739, during the ſame ſpace of time.

April. A cold month for the moſt part, and the principal winds N. and N. W. The ſeventh at night a hurricane from one to four in the morning.

May. Generally fair, and the month con-

concluded hot. The principal winds at ſome point of the E.

It was a healthful ſpring, ſo that few diſeaſes appeared, except the endemial ones, as colds, ſore throats, tumors of the face and jaws, and ophthalmies, to which perhaps might be added a few pleuritic and peripneumonic caſes.

Agues however, which had been rarely ſeen for ſome years paſt, were now pretty frequent; and moreover, the mortal angina deſcribed in the laſt year as raging chiefly in the country, did indeed attack ſome few of our children here, and proved ſuddenly fatal to them: otherwiſe the ordinary ſore throats proved mild enough, as uſual.

SUMMER.

June. The fore and greater part of the month fair, the latter part frequent ſhowers, and ſometimes great changes from ſultry to cold. The principal winds E. N. E. and S. E.

July.

July. Frequent ſhowers the fore and latter part of the month, and the winds variable. From the twelfth to the twenty-ſecond ſerene, and the winds E. and S. E. The month ended cold and wet.

Auguſt. Unſeaſonably wet and windy moſt of the month, and the wind generally W. and S. W. The month concluded ſtormy.

The ſummer-ſeaſon was alſo healthful. I ſaw however ſome ſcrophulous patients to whom the N. and E. winds of laſt ſpring ſeemed to have been very hurtful.

AUTUMN.

September. Generally wet and windy, as the laſt month, and the winds for the moſt part S. W. and W. though ſometimes S. E. and theſe as productive of rain as the S. W. The twenty-ſixth a ſtorm at S. E.

October. Very wet, and ſometimes windy, much like the two former months: the winds variable, and thoſe from the

E.

E. points not lefs attended with rain than the W.

November. Changeable from fair to rain or wind, and fometimes froft, and the winds variable. The fecond, third, fixth, and feventh, ftormy at W. and S. W. The twenty-third and twenty-fourth great floods. The month ended frofty.

The autumnal quarter, though preceded by and attended with much rain and wind, was remarkably more healthy than any of the other feafons (and Huxham obferves the fame thing at Plymouth) fo that in November one of the weekly bills of mortality amounted only to eighteen, about a third of the ufual number. It is indeed no new thing that wet and windy weather fhould prove healthful in thefe countries. The fame obfervation holds good in England, as Wintringham and others conftantly affert.

At the fame time it may be worth while to obferve, that the healthinefs of this year and of the laft fucceeding the great froft in

1739,

1739, 1740, was probably alſo very much promoted by the operation of that froſt, in comminuting and meliorating the ſoil; whence it yielded plenty of good corn, and by the ſucceeding warm ſummers of 1741, 1742, the fruits of the earth were duly maturated, and conſequently wholeſome, and leſs apt to produce a lentor in the blood.

WINTER, 1744, 1745.

December was memorable for three things: 1. A great heighth of the barometer, and at the ſame time very little froſt: 2. A warmth unuſual to the ſeaſon: 3. A great weight of the hygrometer, and predominant moiſture, although very little rain: pleaſant withal, and remarkably healthy. The winds N.W. W. and S.W.

January. Serene partly, but with fogs and froſts interpoſed, and two great falls of ſnow the ninth and twenty-fourth; the wind at S.E. and E. and from the ſnow,

ſnow, with the rain following, very great floods. The principal winds S.E. and N.W.

February. Generally froſty, and ſnow between whiles. The principal winds N.W. N.E. or S.E.

SUMMARY.

Spring very backward, with a prevalence of N. and E. winds.

Summer variable in June and July; in Auguſt very wet and windy.

Autumn rainy.

Winter foggy and partly froſty, eſpecially in February; December warm; great floods in January.

The winter produced but few diſeaſes, except colds, and a few tractable dyſenteries.

In February, a froſty month, the colds became extremely frequent and epidemical, and in ſome few ended in ſudden and fatal peripneumonies.

Some agues alſo (rare of late) made their appearance.

The

The ſum total of burials this year was one thouſand ſeven hundred and five.

SPRING, 1745.

March. A pleaſant and duſty month, for the moſt part warm and ſummer-like, though with a little rain and wind ſometimes interpoſed. The principal winds S. W. then S. E.

April. A cold month, frequent hail, froſt, and ſnow. The principal winds N. E. S. E. S. W. and N. W.

May. Generally very wet and cool, excepting only a very few warm days. The principal winds S. W. rarely S. E. but both attended with moiſture.

Agues, which had been uſhered in laſt year, continued to prevail this ſpring; and in the cold moiſt month of June, they were very irregular in their type.

Our endemial diſeaſes, coughs, anginas, and ophthalmies, did alſo ſometimes appear; and it was obſervable, that ſome of theſe were as frequent in the hot weather ſucceeding

ceeding the cold, as they had been in winter.

SUMMER.

June. Generally cloudy and cold, with frequent ſhowers, and but a few hot days. The principal wind S. W.

July. Generally ſerene and warm. The ſeventeenth a plentiful rain, and a little at the end of the month, and cold. The principal winds N. W. and S. E.

Auguſt. Generally very wet to the twenty-third incluſive, but a few fair days interpoſed. The ſixteenth and ſeventeenth ſtormy at S. W. The month concluded fair. The principal winds S. E. W. and S. W.

July proved generally healthful: at the latter end of the month was a ſudden onſet of cold weather, attended with ophthalmies, anginas, and the ſmall-pox.

In Auguſt was a remarkable increaſe of the articles of fevers, and of the ſmall-pox in the weekly bills, ſo that the laſt on the

the fourth day amounted to twenty-four in a week. Compare the year 1740.

The ſmall-pox were brought to us by a conflux of beggars from the north, occaſioned by the late ſcarcity there, whoſe children, full of the ſmall-pox, were frequently expoſed in our ſtreets.

AUTUMN.

September. Extraordinarily fair and ſummer-like for the moſt part, compenſating in a great meaſure for the late exceſs of rain, and giving a fine opportunity for gathering in the corn. The principal wind S.E. next W.

October. The month began with a hurricane, and the principal weather was wet and windy. Stormy the tenth and eleventh at S.W. and S. The principal wind of the month was S.W.

November. The principal weather was gloomy and foggy, leſs rain and wind than uſual this month: ſome froſt, eſpecially from the fourteenth to the eighteenth. The principal wind was E.

The

The ſummer-like month of September was ſtill fertile in the ſmall-pox, that article in ſome of the weekly bills amounting to twenty-two and twenty-ſeven. They proved frequently fatal this month as well as in Auguſt, and ſeveral died before any maturation.

WINTER, 1745, 1746.

December. The firſt ten days cloudy and foggy, not unpleaſant, with a gentle breeze from the E. thence to the twenty-fourth generally wet and windy, and the wind S.W. then a froſt of a few days, and the month concluded cloudy and mizzling, with a S.E. wind.

January. Very fair and ſummer-like through the firſt fifteen days for the moſt part, and the winds S.W. S.E. and S. The reſt of the month moſtly wet and windy: the winds W. S.W. and S. but it concluded froſty.

February. Generally froſty, and a little ſnow and hail, and ſometimes a little rain. The winds N.E. N.W. and S.W.

SUM-

SUMMARY.

Spring forward in March, but proved backward by the cold of the two following months.

Summer wet.

Autumn variable, ſerene, wet, windy, foggy, and ſome froſt.

Winter open, except the laſt month, which was froſty.

In January fevers were frequent, and proved mortal to ſome*, and more ſo in February.

Coughs were frequent, both in the froſt and on the thaw.

Throughout the year, although comparatively healthy, there were interſperſed, even through the winter, as well as other ſeaſons,

1. Fevers of the low kind, ſometimes with petechiæ, ſometimes with miliary

* Huxham obſerves a bad putrid fever to have prevailed at Plymouth, in December and January.

puſtules,

puftules, though not effentially with either.

2. A more acute fever terminating the fifth, fixth, feventh, or eighth day, with a critical fweat, yet fo that the depuration feemed imperfect: for a relapfe ufually attended, which, however, was commonly carried off by a fecond critical fweat.

The fum total of burials this year was two thoufand two hundred and fixty-five.

SPRING, 1746.

March. The weather was various, according to the common proverb, beginning with froft, fucceeded by hazy and cloudy weather: then from the eighth to the eleventh cold, with fnow and fleet; and this was fucceeded by foft weather and rain, and the month concluded fair and cold. The principal winds S. E. N. E. and N. W.

April. The firft eighteen days alternities of fair and cloudy weather, though moftly cold. The nineteenth two mock-

funs

ſuns appeared, which were followed by a great ſtorm at S. E. The remaining part of the month warmer, with the like changes as above. The principal winds S. E. and N. E.

May. Generally unuſually warm and dry, the thermometer higher than in June and July. The winds S.E. N.E. and E.

Fevers, which had been frequent in winter, continued to be ſo in ſpring, and fatal to ſome.

In May ſeveral inflammations and abſceſſes in the ears occurred; and chincoughs were very epidemic among the children, notwithſtanding the unuſual warmth and ſerenity of the ſeaſon, which however was attended with E. winds. There was alſo among the horſes an epidemical cough, which proved fatal to ſome of them.

SUMMER.

June. Generally cloudy, wet, and cool, and, contrary to cuſtom, wetter and cooler

cooler than May. The winds very variable, the S. W. prevailed.

July. Exceedingly wet and rainy: the ſtreets dirty, as in winter. The principal wind S. W.

Auguſt. Fair weather throughout the month, (except the thirteenth and twenty-firſt, which were rainy,) making compenſation for the redundant moiſture of the two foregoing months, and attended with plenty of all ſorts of grain and fruits, particularly apples. The winds N. W. S. W. and W.

Fevers continued to be frequent through the ſummer, and moſtly acute and inflammatory, as far as I could learn.

AUTUMN.

September. Extremely variable, windy, cloudy, fair, rain, hot, and cold alternately. The winds S. W. N. W. and W.

October. Fine weather for the moſt part: ſome froſt, little rain: the roads dry, and ſprings very low. The winds N. W.

W.

W. N. E. and S. E. From the ſixth to the ſixteenth a moiſt heavy air, with high barometer, which, on the contrary, was low in ſome froſty weather that ſucceeded.

November. The weather and winds were extremely variable; as cloudy, fair, cold, and ſleet, and the twenty-firſt ſultry like ſummer, and ſome ſtorms, particularly the twenty-ſecond at S. W. and W. as it were in conſequence of a previous fermentation. The winds E. N. E. S. E. the foregoing half of the month, thence to the end N. W. S. W. W. and S. E.

Inflammatory fevers continued in September, and were fatal to divers. Some of them became intermittent at the end.

In October coughs were frequent, and much more in November; neither of theſe months were exempt from fevers, which proved mortal to a few.

WINTER, 1746, 1747.

December. The firſt twenty days ſqualls of wind and rain, the winds S. W. and

W.

W. thence to the twenty-eighth cloudy, foggy, and mizzling, and the principal winds S. E. It ended with froſt and ſnow, and S. E. and N. E. winds.

January. Some little froſt at the beginning; but it was generally very wet, and often ſqually. The principal winds S. E.

February. The ſqualls of rain and wind attending the laſt month, continued through the firſt nine days moſtly, and the principal wind S. W. From the fifteenth to the twentieth froſt and a little ſnow, and the winds N. E. and N. Elſe moſtly fair, or gloomy and pleaſant, and the winds S. E. W. and S. W.

SUMMARY.

The firſt part of the ſpring cold, the laſt hot and dry.

A wet ſummer, except the laſt month, which was uncommonly fair.

Autumn very changeable.

Winter wet and windy.

In

Inflammatory fevers, though interſperſed with thoſe of the low kind, continued to be frequent through the winter; and the article of fevers in December, January, and February, was nearly equal to what it had been in the heighth of ſummer. Compare with this the account of laſt winter.

In January coughs were very frequent; and the prevalence of an inflammatory conſtitution appeared from hence, that in the neighbouring county of Kildare, anginas and pleuritic diſorders were now frequent, and often proved fatal in a few days, chiefly among the laborious poor.

The ſum total of burials this year was one thouſand nine hundred and fifty-ſeven.

SPRING, 1747.

March. Dry and froſty for the moſt part, and March duſt in plenty; from the nineteenth almoſt to the end frequent ſnow and ſome ſhowers, and a little wind.

The

The twenty-ſixth windy at S. W. The principal winds at ſome point of the E.

April. Generally fair and dry, and moſtly cool, and void of the uſual ſhowers, except that it was a little cloudy and wet towards the end of the month. The reigning wind S. E.

May. Generally fair and warm weather, and ſhowers frequently interpoſed ; the former attended with S. E. the latter with S. W. winds.

The ſpring, not only the two colder months of March and April, but the warm one of May, were attended with colds, coughs, and inflammatory diſeaſes. In the dry month of April it was particularly obſervable (conſiſtent with Wintringham's obſervation of the effects of the prevalence of the dry E. winds) that the colds proceeded to a more than ordinary degree of inflammation of the membrana Schneideri. Tumors of the face, jaws, and ears, alſo attended this ſpring, and pleuriſies and peripneumonies. Some

aſthma-

aſthmatics ſuffered much. The meazles alſo were frequent through the three ſpring months, being fatal to ſeveral, and the fevers were inflammatory.

SUMMER.

June. The firſt ſix days wet and cool: thence to the twenty-ſecond moſtly fair: thence to the end cloudy and ſhowery. The winds variable.

July. The firſt ſix or ſeven days wet and cloudy, with N. W. and S. W. winds the reſt of the month unuſually ſerene, hot, and dry, for the moſt part, and the reigning winds E. N. E. or S. E.

Auguſt. Remarkably hot and fair, and, contrary to cuſtom, hotter than July, and indeed one of the hotteſt Auguſts in the memory of man. The principal winds S. E. E. or N. E.

The ſummer was generally healthy, eryſipelas's were pretty frequent in July and Auguſt. Several of the fevers in

Auguſt

Auguſt were attended with eruptions on the ſkin, and ſome dogs ran mad.

I met with ſome few of the low fevers in the three ſummer months, interſperſed with thoſe of the acute and inflammatory kind.

AUTUMN.

September introduced as it were a ſudden winter, and the general temperature of the weather was wet. The principal winds N. W. and W.

October. Moſt of the month extraordinarily fair and ſummer-like, ſave that the firſt four days were cloudy and wet, and the month concluded with rain and wind. The principal winds W. S. W. and N. W.

November. The ſummer-like weather of laſt month continued for the moſt part through the firſt fifteen days of this: thence to the end of the month it was alternately wet, windy, and froſty, and concluded with ſleet. The principal winds S. W. and W.

Sep-

September, on the fudden onfet of cold weather, was attended with colds: elfe healthy, though not without fome fevers. October was ftill more healthful, two of the weekly bills only nineteen and twenty; yet it was not without meazles and colds, and fome fporadic fevers.

November alfo exhibited little but colds, except fome few very bad fmall-pox.

WINTER, 1747, 1748.

December. The month began with froft, which was fucceeded by mild, fair weather, or a little gloomy, and fometimes a little rain, and fometimes a little froft through the reft of the month, which concluded with a cold S. E. wind. The principal wind S. E.

January. More warm and ferene than ufual, and often more like April than January, and the thermometer, contrary to cuftom, higher than in December, though not without the gloominefs proper to the feafon interpofed: few frofts, and a few

rainy

rainy days. The principal wind S. E.

February. A good deal of froſt and ſnow, and it was, contrary to cuſtom, colder than January; the eleventh and twenty-ſecond at night, and the twenty-third, rain; elſe generally ſerene and cold, and very frequently froſty. The principal wind S. E.

SUMMARY.

Spring for the moſt part cold.

Summer very hot and dry.

Autumn for the moſt part unuſually fair.

Winter little rain or wind. Froſt in February.

In December the few diſeaſes that fell under my obſervation were of the inflammatory kind, and ſeveral bad ſmall-pox.

In January the unſeaſonably warm weather ſucceeding the cold S. E. wind cloſing the preceding month, was attended with frequent colds and inflammatory diſeaſes, which

which fell heavy on ſome of weak lungs; and the colds of January continued throughout the cold and froſty month of February, and affected the country as well as town.

Total buried this year one thouſand eight hundred and twenty-ſeven.

SPRING, 1748.

March. Alternately wet, windy, fair, cloudy, cold, and ſnow, and mild weather. The winds accordingly variable.

April. The firſt ſeventeen days for the moſt part unſeaſonably cold and dry, and a very backward ſpring: little of falling weather, except hail, which was frequent, and the winds N. W. and N. E. thence to the end of the month warmer, with frequent ſhowers, and the winds generally S. W. and S. E.

May. The rainy weather from the end of laſt month continued at times the firſt eleven days of this: thence to the twenty-firſt moſtly fair: thence to the end of the month

month often cloudy and wet. The principal wind S. W. Often very warm through the month.

The ſpring was healthful, though a few pleuriſies and inflammatory fevers, and ſome few agues were interſperſed. In May the bills of mortality were extremely ſmall, viz. ſeventeen and nineteen; yet, though an extraordinary warmth attended this month, it was not free from tumours of the jaws, and colds.

SUMMER.

June. The cloudy, windy, and cool weather cloſing the laſt month, continued the firſt ſix days of this, and the wind moſtly S. W. thence to the end of the month very warm and dry, and the principal winds S. E. N. E. and E. Some rain at the end.

July. The fair weather was frequently interrupted by ſhowers, and plenty of rain, and ſome winds, eſpecially on the thirteenth, fourteenth, and fifteenth.

The

The thermometer lower than in June, contrary to cuſtom. The principal wind S. W.

Auguſt. The greateſt part of the month fair, and fine harveſt weather, viz. the firſt fifteen days, and the wind N. E. From the fifteenth to the twenty-firſt for the moſt part rainy, and the principal winds W. and S. W. thence to the end of the month fair, and the wind S. E.

June and July were remarkably healthy, the weekly bill in the firſt named month not exceeding ſeventeen and nineteeen, and in July twenty and twenty-one.

Notwithſtanding the exceſſive heat in June, ſome tumours about the face, and colds occurred, otherwiſe very few diſeaſes.

In Auguſt the article of fevers in the weekly bills increaſed; and there were alſo obſervable in this hot month certain tubercles, hot, red, and itching, as from the ſtinging of nettles, the eſſere arabum, attended with no other ſymptom of ſick-

ſickneſs: theſe alſo continued in September.

AUTUMN.

September. The firſt fifteen days moſtly fair, and the principal wind E. thence to the end clouds and rain were interſperſed, and the winds W. S. W. and N. W. ſome days ſultry, and ſome hot winds: a longer protracted ſummer than uſual: the twentieth at night a great fall of rain: the twenty-ninth and thirtieth ſtormy at S. W. and W.

October. The firſt nine days moſtly fair, and ſometimes hazy, and the winds variable: thence to the fourteenth froſty for the moſt part, and the winds N. W. thence to the end frequent rains, particularly the twenty-ſecond at night, and the winds S. E. and S. W. and the month concluded ſtormy at S. W.

November. Generally hazy, ſometimes cloudy and mizzling, rarely ſerene. Uncommonly warm for the ſeaſon: a froſt the twelfth, twentieth, and twenty-firſt. The

The principal winds W. and S. W. It ended windy at S. W.

September was healthy, and more ſo than October, about the ninth day of which laſt we had, after a long ſeries of uncommonly fair weather, a ſudden onſet as of winter, with froſt and rain, which was followed by an increaſe of the number of fevers, which were at leaſt partly inflammatory, and ſome quinzies, and ſome bad meazles; and yet though the ſeaſon was ſickly, the diſeaſes were not mortal: and ſeveral of the fevers that occurred this month were happily terminated by ſweat the fifth or ſixth day.

The warm month of November was alſo generally healthy.

WINTER, 1748, 1749.

December. Windy at S. W. the greateſt part of the month, and not much rain. The fifteenth a deep ſnow, and in the night a ſtorm, and the ſixteenth a great fall of ſnow and ſleet.

Janu-

January. Windy at S. W. and W. through the greateſt part of the month: frequent ſtorms, eſpecially in the nights, particularly the twenty-ſixth. A good deal of rain and floods: the eleventh and twelfth at night lightning. Some little froſt, ſnow, and ſleet, eſpecially near the end, but of no duration.

February. Windy at times at S. W. the firſt nine days: thence to the ſeventeenth a remarkable calmneſs and ſerenity, ſucceeding our long continued ſtorms, and the winds ſhifted to S. E. thence to the end cloudy and wet, and the winds continued S. E.

SUMMARY.

Spring variable, and pretty ſeaſonable.

Summer generally warm and dry.

Autumn uncommonly warm and ſummer-like.

Winter windy and warm.

The whole winter quarter was remarkably healthful, ſo that little occurred except

cept a few coughs. What few fevers I met with were chiefly of the low kind.

Total buried this year one thoufand five hundred and thirty.

SPRING, 1749.

March. The firft thirteen days rainy and warm: this was fucceeded by dry and fharp weather, which lafted more or lefs to the end of the month: near the end it was lefs cold, and there was more rain. The twenty-fixth a great flood. The principal wind S. E.

April. An unufually cold month for the moft part, a good deal of rain, and fome hail: it concluded fair and warm. The principal winds S. E. and S. W.

May. The firft nine days for the moft part cold weather, like that of March, and the fifth a great fall of fnow. From the tenth to the twentieth a feries of fair and very warm weather, thence to the end, and efpecially fince the appearance of a mock-fun on the twenty-third, it grew cold

cold and winter-like, withrain and hail. The winds variable.

Notwithſtanding the great viciſſitudes of the weather, the ſpring was healthful. Coughs and colds were very frequent in March, and ſome of theſe appeared in May on the warm weather ſucceeding the late unſeaſonably cold. Some agues alſo attended this ſpring, and ſome dyſenteries.

SUMMER.

June. The firſt eighteen days cold and winter-like, yet alternately fair and cloudy during this period. A parhelion or mock-ſun appeared the ſixteenth, which was followed by ſtormy weather. The wind during the aforeſaid period chiefly N. W. From the nineteenth to the end generally fair and warm, and the winds S. W. and W.

July. A little windy at the beginning: the firſt thirteen days for the moſt part fair. From the fourteenth to the end alternately fair and ſhowers. The eighteenth

teenth and twenty-fourth much rain. The principal wind S. W.

Auguft. The foregoing half of the month it was often cloudy, wet, cold, and winter-like; the latter half of the month generally fair, and fine harveft-weather: the winds S. W. and N. W. The twenty-third and thirtieth much rain: the month ended cold and fair.

The fummer in general was very healthy: aguifh diforders were the chief which were frequent both in town and country, promoted, as it feems, by the winter-like and changeable ftate of the weather.

AUTUMN.

September. A hafty onfet of winter, as it were; the firft twenty days moftly cloudy, a good deal of rain, and frequently cold, almoft to froft: the reft of the month partly fair, and partly hazy. The principal winds N. W. S. W. and W.

October. Dry and mild, except the firft fix days, which were wet and windy:

elfe

elſe hazy and pleaſant, and a little froſt ſometimes; but the month concluded warm. The principal winds N. W. S. W. and W.

November. A fine mild month, as the former, moſtly warm and calm; rarely froſty, as the ſixth and twenty-ſeventh; rain the fifth, ſeventh, and eighth; a little windy the twenty-fourth and twenty-fifth. The winds W. S. W. and S. E.

The autumn was not productive of many diſeaſes: ſome pleuriſies occurred in October, and coughs were frequent in October and November.

WINTER 1749, 1750.

December. The mild weather of the two preceding months continued through a conſiderable part of this: the firſt eight days for the moſt part gloomy and pleaſant: the ninth and tenth a glut of rain, which was ſucceeded by frequent froſts and cold weather, until near the end of the month, which was mild. The principal wind S W.

January. The greateſt part of the month

month was mild, being alternately fair, hazy, cloudy, and foggy, with a little rain and wind, and ſome ſlight froſts, and ſometimes warm weather like ſpring: the principal wind S. W. S. E. and S. From the twenty-fifth to the end wet and windy, and the principal wind S. W.

February. Very windy, frequently ſtormy and wet: the reigning wind S. W. next W. a few ſerene days: it concluded with ſnow and froſt.

SUMMARY.

Spring cold.

Summer partly cold and winter-like.

Autumn for the moſt part mild, warm, and dry.

Winter mild and open.

The winter was healthy; ſo that little but the endemial diſeaſes of the country, viz. coughs and defluxions, were frequent in December and January. In February ſeveral agues appeared from the beginning to the end of the month.

Total buried this year one thouſand eight hundred and ſeventeen.

SPRING.

SPRING, 1750.

March. The foregoing half of the month, eſpecially the firſt ten days, pleaſant and mild, the reſt of the month windy, wet, and hail and froſt interſperſed. The principal winds N. W. S. W. and W.

April. Alternately fair and cloudy, with a little rain interſperſed, and ſometimes hail: it was frequently cold, and ſometimes froſty, but ended mild. The principal winds N. E. S. E. and N. W.

May. Generally fair and extremely dry, and ſometimes froſty in the mornings. The principal winds N. E. E. and S. E. The month concluded with ſhowers, and N. W. and ſoutherly winds. A backward ſpring.

Agues, which had begun in February, were the prevailing diſeaſe in March, and they were very irregular.

March and April were not exempt from continual fevers, partly of the low, nervous,

vous, and petechial kind, and partly partaking of the intermittent. The ſharp weather in April proved pernicious to ſome conſumptive perſons; and colds were frequent this month, and in May became very epidemic, promoted, no doubt, by the long continued eaſterly winds: alſo ſeveral pleuriſies occurred in May.

SUMMER.

June. Frequent rains, and ſometimes very cold, and the hygrometer heavier than in May. The principal winds S. W. and N. W. nevertheleſs ſo changeable was the temperature of the weather this month, that from the 17th to the 21ſt it was the hotteſt weather in the memory of man; and Fahrenheit's thermometer roſe to ſeventy-ſix, which is as high as it is noted to have riſen at any time in lord Anſon's voyage round the world, though in London it once roſe to ſeventy-eight.

July. The firſt ſeven days it was frequently cloudy and wet: from the eighth

to

to the twelfth fair, and exceſſively hot, Farenheit's thermometer again mounting to ſeventy-ſix. From the twelfth to the twenty-ſecond cloudy and wet; thence to the end frequent ſhowers: the dog-days cold. The principal wind S. W. and the hygrometer heavier than in June.

Auguſt. A winterly month: the firſt half of it ſcarce a day without rain, the latter half it cleared up a little; but ſtill rain was interſperſed, and the dog-days were remarkably cold, though the month concluded ſultry. The principal wind S. W.

The ſummer-quarter, notwithſtanding its predominant moiſture, and the great changes from extreme heat to cold, appeared by all obſervations to have been remarkably healthy.

Some aguiſh diſorders attended July and Auguſt, and thoſe very irregular. July exhibited ſome chin-coughs, and Auguſt ſome coughs; and I think he muſt have been ſceptical who would deny the

above

above defcribed ftate of the weather to have had any influence on the difeafes.

AUTUMN.

September. Pleafant weather, calm, fair, and gloomy; fometimes warm like fummer, compenfating as it were for the bad fummer; and the harveft proved good. The fecond, twelfth, and fourteenth rainy, elfe very little rain. The winds moftly at fome point of the N. or E.

October. Generally cool, with cloudy and hazy weather by turns, and fometimes rain and fnow, which fell in gluts at once, particularly the feventh and tenth; and the twenty-third at night was a vaft fall of hail and fnow, which was followed by a very fmart froft, and, what is uncommon fo early in the feafon, lafting almoft to the end of the month. The principal winds E. S. E. and N. W.

November. Frequent frofts, with fogs and little wind: hazy and ferene by turns.

The

The fourth and twenty-ninth at night a great glut of rain. The twenty-ninth and thirtieth a ſtorm at S. W. The principal wind N. W.

Some choleras appeared about the beginning of September, which otherwiſe was a healthy month, as was alſo the greateſt part of October, until the memorable fall of ſnow the twenty-third, which was ſucceeded by a greater frequency of colds both in the city and country, and fevers became a little more frequent; and with the continuation of the cold in November our colds were alſo increaſed, and a ſomewhat more ſickly ſeaſon attended: and I apprehend that he muſt be more than ſceptical who would in this further inſtance, deny the influence of the weather on diſeaſes; and, on the contrary, I would take upon me to caution valetudinarians to beware of all great and ſudden changes in the weather, and uſe the neceſſary precautions.

WIN-

WINTER, 1750, 1751.

December. The firſt five days windy and wet; then warm, ſpring-like weather, and the thermometer conſiderably higher than in November: foggy and mizzling afterwards, and a ſlight froſt near the end, but of no duration. The principal winds S. E. S. and S. W.

January. Extremely variable weather, cloudy, ſerene, wet, warm, and cold, and frequent froſts with ſnow, eſpecially at the latter end of the month. The winds alſo variable. The ſixteenth at night a violent ſtorm from twelve to three in the morning followed, by a great fall of rain.

February. The firſt eight days fair and froſty, with E. and S. E. winds, then windy and wet, and ſometimes froſt and hail, rarely ſerene.

The principal winds the reſt of the month S. W. and N. W. The twenty-fifth at night a great fall of rain, and a violent ſtorm.

SUM-

SUMMARY.

Spring cold, dry, and backward.

Summer (excepting a few exceſſively hot days) cold, moiſt, and winter-like.

Autumn variable, mild at the beginning, froſty after.

Winter (except December, which was warm) exhibited a good deal of froſt and ſnow.

Very few diſeaſes occurred in December. In January our endemial coughs and defluxions made their appearance. In February, with the continued cold of the ſeaſon, thoſe diſorders alſo continued, and there was a little increaſe in the bills of mortality.

About the middle or latter end of December the moſt epidemic and univerſally ſpreading diſeaſe among horſes that any one living remembered, made its appearance in Dublin, which ſeems to have been nearly analogous to the influenza and catarrhal fever which ſeized mankind in the years

years 1737 and 1743; but now peculiarly attacked the horſes in their turn, as may appear by a comparriſon of their reſpective hiſtories, of the latter of which here follows a ſummary one.

It had appeared in England in November, and ſpread through all England almoſt in an inſtant; and towards the end of the month began to abate. It raged in Denmark at the ſame time: but it did not reach our horſes in Dublin till its decline in England at the time before mentioned, having probably been imported, and was nearly of the ſame duration here as in England: however, it affected the horſes in Munſter and Ulſter almoſt, if not quite, as ſoon as in Dublin; and there was ſcarce an inſtance of a horſe in town or country but had it.

It ſeized them like a violent cold, with heavineſs, loſs of appetite, cough, and laborious breathing, and then a profuſe running at the noſe and mouth, of a digeſted or thick yellow greeniſh matter; upon which they grew better.

In England, as well as here, it did not prove very mortal, though ſome died of it. In our barracks, out of one hundred and forty-four horſes, I heard of but three that died.

The moſt ſucceſsful method was to keep them warm, and give them the white maſh, or bran ſcalded with water, and walk them about a little daily.

The death of our horſes in the city was imputed rather to the uſe of medicines, and too high a diet, than to any malignity in the diſeaſe; for it was obſervable, that very few died in the country, and particularly none that were kept at graſs. It vaniſhed about the middle of January *.

The ſum total of burials this year was two thouſand and eighty-eight.

SPRING, 1751.

March A windy, wet, and cold month,

* In the year 1699, after a warm February and March, April was very cold, and there was a general cough among horſes all over England, France, &c: ſcarce one eſcaped, yet not one died. SHORT's Chronological Hiſtory of the Weather and Seaſons.

frequent

frequent hail, and ſome froſt and ſnow. The principal winds W. and S. W.

April. A cold month for the moſt part, with a prevalence of N. E. winds: ſome few days warm and pleaſant: the rains not ſo frequent, but more in gluts than uſual, v. g. the tenth, twelfth, fourteenth, fifteenth, were rainy; elſe little rain.

May. The firſt half of the month alternately fair and cloudy, ſometimes windy, ſhowers frequently of hail, and moſtly cold. The latter part of the month for the moſt part fair and warm. The tenth, twelfth, ſixteenth, and ſeventeenth, rainy. The principal winds N. W. S. E. and S. W.

Irregular agues were frequent in March, as were alſo tumours of the face, jaws, and throat: agues alſo continued to be frequent in April, both in the city and in ſeveral parts of the country.

Coughs alſo were frequent; and many in chronical diſorders of the breaſt were

worſe

worſe and weaker in this cold month than they had been in the middle of winter, and many of the conſumptive died: otherwiſe it was far from being a ſickly ſeaſon.

In May the prevailing morbid conſtitution was much like that of the two preceding months, coughs being ſtill as frequent as in winter, and the article of continual fevers very moderate.

SUMMER.

June. The fair and warm weather continued moſt of the firſt twelve days of this month, with S. E. and N. E. winds. The twelfth day remarkably hot, and the thermometer at ſeventy-ſix; but this was of no continuance: a great drought attended moſt of the month, notwithſtanding that S. W. winds were frequently interpoſed: the latter part of the month cool, with E. and ſometimes S. W. winds.

July. Frequent and plentiful rains: few days entirely free from rain. The principal winds S. W. N. W. and S. E.

Au-

August. The firſt nineteen days for the moſt part rainy, thence to the end of the month generally fair. The principal wind S. W.

This ſummer was very remarkably healthy, the article of fevers unuſually low; and thoſe few that did occur ſeem to have been of the low kind, and ſome agues *.

AUTUMN.

September. A wet month, few fair days: a great glut of rain the twentieth, twenty-firſt, twenty-ſecond, and great floods. The principal winds S. W. W. and N. W.

* The like healthineſs alſo was obſervable in London: for from the ſixth to the thirteenth of Auguſt, there died but two hundred and twenty-four, which is ſaid to be the leaſt number that have died in the ſame ſpace of time ſince the year 1665. An ingenious obſerver in the London Magazine, imputes this healthineſs of the ſeaſon to the equability of the temper of the air, manifeſted by the thermometer and barometer, together with the moiſture of the ſeaſon, as being the leaſt productive of diſeaſes in England; which alſo holds good here.

Octo-

October. Fair and pleafant for the moft part, and the wind S.E. flight frofts pretty frequent: the twenty-fifth and twenty-fixth a glut of rain, with a N.E. wind, and the month concluded with a fmart froft.

November. Hazy and foggy for the moft part, and a little froft at the beginning and near the conclufion: the winds moftly S.W. and W. The fixteenth at night, feventeenth, and twenty-firft ftormy. The fourteenth, twenty-third at night, and twenty-fourth rainy.

The autumn alfo was healthy; fo that little memorable occurred, except that colds became frequent in October on the eafterly winds and flight frofts, and coughs attended the whole month of November, fome of which were fevere.

WINTER, 1751, 1752.

December. Hazy, foggy, cloudy, or mizzling; fometimes a little rain and fome frofts, efpecially the thirteenth and four-

teenth

teenth days, and at the end. The twentieth at night a great fall of rain. The principal winds N. W. and S. E.

January. Hazy, dark, and cloudy weather, the ſun rarely appearing: frequent rains, particularly the ninth, tenth, thirteenth, and fourteenth days, moſtly with a S. E. wind. Snow the nineteenth and twenty-fourth, which was more frequent in the country.

February. For the moſt part pleaſant, fair, and moderate, with a high barometer. The twelfth and fourteenth at night rain, as alſo the twenty-firſt. The fourteenth at night and the twenty-ſixth ſtormy. The principal winds S. W. and N. W.

SUMMARY.

Spring cold.

Summer wet.

Autumn variable.

Winter hazy and cloudy, little froſt: a fair February.

The winter was healthy, particularly December; wherein, in the article of fever

in

in the bills of mortality there was none twice in the month, a great rarity: coughs however, our endemial diſeaſe, prevailed greatly and chiefly; and ſeveral little inflammations on the face, eyes, and gums, occurred: the meazles alſo were frequent.

The bills of mortality increaſed a little in January, though ſtill low; but coughs were ſtill frequent, beſides a few ſore throats and ophthalmies.

In February the ſum total of the bills was ſomewhat greater than in the two preceding months, though ſtill but moderate; but the meazles were very epidemic.

Total buried this year two thouſand and thirty.

N. B. In December and January, being about the ſame time as laſt year, there prevailed again among the horſes an epidemical catarrh, being attended with a running at the eyes, and heavineſs, with a tumor of the head, limbs, and ſometimes ſcrotum, not ſo general as laſt year, though ſome few died.

SPRING,

SPRING 1752.

March. Cold and dry for the moſt part, ſometimes windy, frequent froſts, ſome hail and ſnow. The principal winds N. W. and N. E.

April. For the moſt part extremely dry and cold: few ſhowers, and thoſe frequently of hail. The principal winds N. E. E. S. E. or N. W.

May. A moiſt, dropping month: a few warm days, eſpecially from the ninth to the thirteenth, as alſo the twenty-ſeventh. The principal winds S. E. and E.

The ſpring was moderately healthful. The meazles, as in February, continued to be very epidemic in March and April: ſome few agues appeared in April: coughs were frequent in April and May, and ſore throats were frequent in May.

The peſtilential angina (of which ſee the account above A. D. 1743) made ſome appearance in April, in the neigh-

bour-

bourhood of the city, particularly about Kilgobben and Kilternan, making great havock among the children, of whom one, aged two years and a half, died in eight or ten hours after the feizure.

SUMMER.

June. The prevailing weather was cloudy, wet, cool, and winter-like: few fair and warm days. The principal winds S. W.

July. Exceffively wet, but very few days quite free from rain, which fometimes fell in great abundance, particularly the twenty fixth. The principal wind N. W.

Auguft. Cloudy and wet: much rain the eleventh and twenty-fourth at night, and the twenty-fifth day. The principal wind S. W.

The fummer-quarter was as remarkable for being healthful as it was for being exceffively wet. Some fmall-pox occurred, agreeable to Huxham's obfervation of their being

being feffile, and not duly maturating in wet feafons.

AUTUMN.

September. The moift weather of laft month continued by intervals through the greateft part of this: it was frequently windy. The principal wind S. W. but it concluded fair, with an E. wind.

October. A fine, mild month, moderate, ferene, and foggy alternately; the winds S. E. and S. W. The eighth at night, and the thirteenth at night, a great fall of rain.

November. Hazy, fair, foggy, and fome flight frofts, and fometimes a little windy; fome rains, not frequent, but in great gluts, as the fourth, fifth, ninth, and twenty-fourth; the tenth a great fall of fnow. The principal wind S. W.

The autumn in general was healthful. Coughs became more frequent, efpecially fince the great fall of fnow the tenth of November, and feveral dyfenteries appeared,

WIN-

WINTER, 1752, . 1753.

December. Moftly hazy and foggy, little wind: frequent frofts, efpecially the latter part of the month. The feventeenth at night a ftorm, fucceeded by a great fall of rain, and fnow the eighteenth at night. The principal winds W. S. W. and N. W.

January. Foggy and frequent frofts, a few ferene days, a little fnow, and frequent rains. The principal winds S. W. W. and S. E.

February. Froft and fnow very frequent, and great rains between whiles. The twelfth a great fnow, the fixteenth and feventeenth ftormy. The principal winds S. E. W. and S. W. The month ended fair, with N. E. winds.

SUMMARY.

Spring cold and dry, excepting a moift May.

Summer extremely wet.

Autumn

Autumn moderate and dry.

Winter frofty, with fnow and frequent rains.

Coughs were extremely frequent and epidemic, and were indeed the chief reigning difeafe through the three winter months, befides a few dyfenteries.

Total buried this year one thoufand eight hundred and forty-four. In London twenty thoufand four hundred eighty-five. In both places a lefs number than ufual of late.

SPRING, 1753.

March. Moftly dry the firft eleven days, with S. E. and N. E. winds; the reft of the month wet, fo that there was fcarce a day without rain, and fometimes hail and flight frofts. The fifteenth, fixteenth, and twenty-fifth at night great falls of rain. The principal winds through the latter and greater part of the month S. W. and frequent fqualls.

April. The foregoing half of the month alternately fair and fhowery as ufual,

ufual, and hail frequent, with N. E. and N. W. winds: the latter part of the month warm, with more frequent W. and S. W. winds, and fhowers interfperfed; and it concluded windy.

May. Serene moftly the firft nine days, and the principal wind at fome point of the E. thence to the twenty-firft cloudy and cold, with frequent fhowers, and the wind N. W. thence to the end warm, ferene, and very pleafant, with E. winds.

Coughs and colds, which had been very frequent in winter, continued through the three fpring months. In April the chief difeafes attacked the cheft, and fome of a tabid difpofition fuffered. The fame month a violent raucedo and tumour of the jaws was epidemic among fome young children in the fuburbs.

Several irregular intermittent diforders appeared in March, and a few in May, when alfo fome fore throats attended.

SUMMER.

June. The firſt half of the month was for the moſt part fair and hot; the laſt half, it was frequently cold, cloudy, and wet, with N.W. winds: elſe S. E. S. W. and N. E.

July. The foregoing half of the month wet, ſo that ſcarce a day was free from rain, and the principal winds S. E. and N. W. The reſt of the month moſtly fair, and the winds N. W. and N. E.

Auguſt. Frequent rains the firſt half of the month, particularly a great fall the fourth at night and the fifteenth. The remainder of the month moſtly dry, fair, ſometimes gloomy, cloudy, and cool. The principal winds W. and S. W.

Coughs and colds continued to be very frequent in June, not only on the change of weather from warm to cold, but even in, as well as after the warm weather.

The article of fevers was but very ſmall in our bills during the three ſummer-

months;

months; however, I met with ſeveral in which the time of the criſis was various, viz. in three the fifth day; in two the fourteenth day; in two others the ninth. In one the ſeventh, with relapſes; in another the twelfth; in another the nineteenth. In one the twenty-third, which was of the petechial kind, and fatal.

AUTUMN.

September. A fine, dry, ſummer-like month, though it ended a little windy and wet, with S. W. winds, which elſe were variable.

October. Moſtly dry throughout the month, and ſeveral warm and ſummer-like days, and there was but little rain, even with the S. W. winds, which were the predominant. The eighth at night and ſixteenth only rainy. The month concluded foggy, inclining to froſt, with N. E. and N. winds.

November. A little wet and windy at the beginning, afterwards frequent froſt through-

throughout the month. The firſt, twenty-fifth, and twenty-ſixth wet and windy: the twenty-ſecond and twenty-third warm. Winds S. W. W. N. W. and N.

Fevers were not unfrequent in September, in the city; and in the ſuburbs, particularly at Kilmainham, but not mortal. Among nine of them in different ages, which occurred to me, the time of the termination varied from the fifth to the eighth or ninth, tenth, twelfth, fourteenth, ſeventeenth, and thirtieth day.

In October the fevers were of ſhorter duration, as far as I obſerved, terminating the ſeventh, eighth, and fourteenth day: on the change to cold weather colds were frequent.

In November coughs continued to be epidemical, and ſome fevers attended, which terminated in fourteen and ſeven days; but more in fourteen.

WINTER, 1753, 1754.

December. The firſt nine days cold, foggy, and froſty, and the wind N. W. thence

thence to the twenty-ſixth frequent rains, and more than had fallen for ſeveral months paſt, The winds W. and S. W. the end it was froſty again, with N. W. and N. E. winds.

January. The firſt twenty-four days cloudy, with frequent rains, particularly the fourth at night, and the fourteenth and fifteenth at night: great inundations in the country; the winds S. W. and W. The tenth a ſtorm at S. W. From the twenty-fifth to the end a ſmart froſt, with N. W. winds.

February. The firſt eight days cold, and frequent ſnow and ſleet, the reſt of the month viciſſitudes of cloudy, fair, and rainy weather. The twelfth ſtormy and rainy. The principal winds S. W. and N. W.

SUMMARY.

Spring ſeaſonable, excepting a wet March.

Sum-

Summer wet, not above one half ſummer-like.

Autumn fair and dry, ending froſty.

Winter rainy, and great floods, with froſts interpoſed.

Coughs and diſorders of the lungs were frequent through the three winter-months. January was fatal to ſeveral of the conſumptive.

February exhibited a greater number of fevers than December or January, in which alſo the lungs were remarkably attacked. Of the ſeveral fevers that occurred to me this quarter, the days of termination were the fifth, ſixth, ſeventh, ninth, (eleventh, which was of the petechial kind and fatal) the ſeventeenth, nineteenth, twenty-firſt, and twenty-third.

Total buried this year one thouſand eight hundred and twenty-five.

SPRING, 1754.

March. The firſt nine days alternately ſerene, gloomy, and foggy; the reſt of the

the month was for the moſt part unuſually cold, except the twenty-third day, which was mild: frequent froſts, hail, and ſnow. The principal wind N. E.

April. The firſt fourteen days moſtly fair, and a few clouds and ſhowers interſperſed, and the winds variable: thence to the end very cold, and frequent hail, ſnow, and ſleet, and the wind moſtly N. W. thence to the end for the moſt part fair, and the winds. N. W. E. and S. E.

May. Alternately fair, cloudy, and ſhowery, and the principal wind at ſome point of the E. It ended fair, with E. winds.

Diſorders of the breaſt chiefly prevailed in the extraordinarily cold month of March; and April exhibited chiefly the ſame ſort of diſeaſes, viz. coughs and aſthmas; and the conſumptive ſuffered greatly.

This ſpring agues were frequent in the counties of Kilkenny and Carlow, though rare in Dublin.

Of

Of the continuals that occurred to me, one had a critical ſweat the fifth day, another the fourteenth, a third the fifteenth, and a fourth died the ſeventeenth day.

SUMMER.

June extremely wet and windy for the moſt part, few days without rain, great floods at the middle of the month. The principal winds W. and N. W.

July. Moſty fair the firſt ſix days, the reſt of the month wet and very cold, eſpecially in the nights. The principal winds W. and N. W.

Auguſt. The wet weather continued the firſt eight days; the reſt of the month moſtly fair, and ſometimes hot; but it concluded cool, and a little windy. The principal winds N. W. S. E. and E.

I can ſay nothing from obſervation concerning the diſeaſes of the ſummer-quarter, having ſpent it in retirement in the country for the recovery of my own health; but was well aſſured that it was healthy, ſave

ſave that at the latter end of Auguſt fevers became more frequent, and proved fatal to ſeveral.

AUTUMN.

September. Fine harveſt-weather, fair and pleaſant, and frequently warm, like ſummer: the tenth and twenty-ſixth at night rain; the principal wind S. E.

October. Fair weather continued to prevail throughout the month: from the eighth to the eighteenth, and the twenty-third, twenty-fourth, twenty-fifth windy: the ſixteenth, early in the morning, a great ſtorm: the fifteenth and thirtieth much rain: the nineteenth, twentieth, and twenty-firſt ſultry, as in ſummer, with a heavy hygrometer, and the thermometer higher than in May. Winds W. S. W. and N. W.

November. Moſtly fair throughout the month, and ſome ſummer-like days, though ſometimes cloudy and foggy: the ſixth and ninth at night rain, and near the end a ſmart

ſmart froſt for four days. The principal winds N. W. and S. E.

The diſeaſes of this autumn, being a ſummer-like ſeaſon ſucceeding a wet ſummer, were chiefly thoſe of the lower belly, which ſeemed to be owing to indigeſtion, and eating fruit not well ripened; whence pains and tenſions, and a conſiderable number of dyſenteries: alſo ſome coughs and catarrhs.

Beſides theſe, there occurred alſo during the three autumnal months, here and there, a certain fever which proved fatal to ſeveral. An obſervator of the weather and diſeaſes in London during the ſame time takes notice of a dangerous remittent fever, although not very frequent, which occurred there alſo, in which bleeding was hurtful. It is probable that ours was akin to theirs, and owing to the ſame general cauſes.

The chief of thoſe that fell under my obſervation ran out to three weeks, and one of them to ſix: the heat not great, the attack mild and deceitful.

WIN-

WINTER, 1754, 1755.

December. The foregoing half of the month was alternately cloudy, fair, wet, windy, and ſometimes foggy, and the principal wind S. W. The eighth at night a great fall of rain: the latter half of the month for the moſt part hazy and foggy, rarely a little ſpitting, moſtly cool, and the principal wind S. E.

January. For the moſt part dry, cold, and froſty, and the winds S. E. N. E. and E. ſometimes S. W. It concluded with a ſmart froſt.

February. For the moſt part froſty throughout the month, and the winds S. E. E. and N. E. the nineteenth rainy; the twenty-firſt, twenty-ſecond, twenty-third, a good deal of ſnow: it ended cloudy and cool.

SUMMARY.

Spring partly temperate, partly cold.
Summer wet.
Autumn fair and ſummer-like.
Winter froſty.

In December and January appeared ſeveral dyſenteries, the reliques of the foregoing autumn: alſo among ſome children a cough, with fever and eruptions in the ſkin, as in the meazles.

In February coughs, colds, and diſorders of the lungs were very frequent; and throughout the three winter-months a fever was frequent, which proved fatal to ſeveral, that article in February riſing to almoſt double the uſual number.

It attacked all ages, and ſeems to have been of the low depreſſed kind, and commonly attended with miliary or other puſtules, the time of the eruption of which was various, as uſual. The criſis in thoſe that fell under my obſervation was for the moſt part before the fourteenth or fifteenth day, and in ſeveral on the nineteenth, twentieth, or twenty-firſt; and although others terminated ſooner, and ſome died in a few days confinement, there was great reaſon to think that theſe laſt had a lurking fever ſeveral days before,

fore, which were not taken into the reckoning.

It feems to have been a continuation of the fever of the laft autumn, and common to Dublin and London both in autumn and winter.

N. B. The gangrenous fore throat of 1743 attacked fome children in this city, and proved fatal to feveral: one of them was thirteen years old.

Total buried this year one thoufand eight hundred and ninety-feven, according to one account; but according to another perhaps more accurate, one thoufand feven hundred and thirty-two.

SPRING, 1755.

March. Mild weather, fnow or froft rare, but frequent rains throughout the month, and rarely a day without rain, though no great glut of rain. It ended warm amd windy. The principal winds S. W. N. W. S. E. and N. E.

April. Wet, much like the preceding month, not many days without rain: fome fine weather, but rarely, and the month concluded cold. The principal wind. S. W

May. The firſt ſixteen days alternately fair and cloudy, and often rainy; moſtly cool, ſome hail: thence to the end of the month moſtly fair, warm, and pleaſant: the thirtieth day rainy: The principal winds W. and N. W.

The bills in March were higher than for a long time paſt; but this ſeems to have proceeded rather from conſumptions and decays by age than from acute diſeaſes: and accordingly many coughs and conſumptions occurred in March and April, although wet and mild months, but which had been preceded by a ſevere winter, which probably laid the foundation for the fatality.

Fevers of the eruptive kind, and ſome of them miliary, appear to have been common to us and London in March and April.

Of four continuals that occurred this ſpring, two terminated the fourteenth, another the twentieth, a fourth the fifth day. In

In May, whilſt the bills were lower than in the two preceding months, a conſiderable number of cutaneous diſorders, and ſeveral eryſipelas's attended; and colds were frequent the firſt half of the month.

SUMMER.

June. Excepting the firſt four days, which were fair, with E. winds, the greater part of the reſt of the month was cloudy, and frequently wet: the ſeventh, thirteenth, nineteenth, and twenty-ninth, rainy. The winds variable.

July. A very wet month, few days without clouds or rain: the ſecond at night, the fifth at night, the eighth at night, the fifteenth at night, and the nineteenth and twenty-firſt days much rain: it concluded fair. The winds N. W. S. W. and W.

Auguſt. The foregoing half of the month alternately cloudy and fair, the latter part more cloudy and hazy: cool in general:

general: the eighteenth and twenty-eighth at night a confiderable fall of rain. The winds N.W. and W.

Eryfipelas's, which are obferved above to have attended May, continued to be frequent in fummer.

Fevers, feveral of them of the petechial kind, were frequent in fummer, particularly in Auguft, though more favourable than of late: the times of the termination of thofe that occurred to my obfervation this quarter were various, viz. the fourth, fixth, tenth, eleventh, twelfth, fourteenth, twentieth, twenty-firft and twenty-third days; and two on the feventh, and one of the low kind, with all the marks of fever, except quicknefs of pulfe, but with diarrhœa and cold fweats, ran out to a month, and the patient recovered.

I met with two intermittents in Auguft, and three obftinate rheumatifms; and fome of the patients, although not old, were from thence deprived of the ufe of their limbs.

1. Did

1. Did not the long continued moiſture of the ſpring and ſummer evidently promote the diſorders prevailing this ſummer, particularly the low putrid fevers, and rheumatiſms?

2. As I obſerved the accounts here given of the prevailing fevers this and laſt ſpring, as well as laſt year, to have agreed nearly to thoſe publiſhed concerning the reigning diſeaſes in London at the ſame time, is not a mutual correſpondence between phyſicians worthy to be recommended?

AUTUMN.

September. Generally cloudy and frequent rains: gluts of rain the firſt and twenty-eighth at night, and cool. The fifteenth and ſixteenth ſummer-like days, elſe very little harveſt-weather; and the month concluded wet and ſtormy. The principal wind S. W.

October. The beginning of the month a little windy, then fair weather and

frequent

frequent frosts to the eighteenth: the rest of the month fair, foggy, and hazy: a fine dry month, and some warm summer-like days. The winds variable.

November. Variable, viz. hazy, windy, and cloudy, the first week: then frost, hail, and snow, to the twelfth. The thirteenth and fourteenth much rain and floods; wet and windy to the twenty-fourth. It concluded frosty. Winds W. N.W. and S.W.

It was a healthy autumn, though not exempt from fevers; but much more rare in the fine dry month of October, than in September and November.

Some hemiplegias attended October, and indeed this disease has for some months past been more frequent in Dublin, and some parts of the country, than for many years before, perhaps from the excessive moisture of the seasons: these and a few coughs and colds, and fifteen fevers, made up the complement of my observations this quarter, of which fifteen two died:

died: of theſe ſome were petechial, ſome inflammatory, but both bore bleeding, and the firſt without regard to the effloreſcences on the ſkin. The time of the criſis of theſe fevers, which attacked both children and the middle aged and elderly, was as various as their ages, habits, and the weather attending; and accordingly happened on the fifth, ſixth, ſeventh, eighth, eleventh, twelfth, fourteenth, ſixteenth, twentieth, twenty-fourth, twenty-ſixth, and on the forty-ſecond, in a man in the decline of life.

WINTER, 1755, 1756.

December. Alternately rain and froſt, and ſometimes ſnow: the eleventh, fourteenth, and fifteenth, gluts of rain: the twenty-fourth at night ſtormy. Winds S. W. W. and N. W.

January. Rain through the greateſt part of the month, from the eighth to the eleventh, and from the nineteenth to the twenty-fifth windy. The ſixteenth a ſmart froſt. Winds S. W. W. and N. W.

Fe-

February. Windy through great part of the month, and moſtly at S. W. The twelfth at night a hurricane, which did ſome damage. The windy weather was ſucceeded by a little froſt, then foggy and fair weather. Winds S. W. and W.

SUMMARY.

Spring wet.

Summer wet.

Autumn wet, except October.

Winter wet.

It was a healthy winter, and particularly the windy month of February afforded abundance of leiſure. Our endemial diſeaſes, coughs, chin-coughs, ſwelled jaws, were the chief; and diſorders of the lungs, which proved fatal to ſeveral.

The few fevers that I heard of during this winter-quarter, which were partly petechial, and partly inflammatory, were for the moſt part mortal, on the fifth or ſixth, the fourteenth or fifteenth, ſixteenth, and twentieth days.

Total

Total buried this year two thouſand and two; or, from a more accurate account, one thouſand eight hundred and ninety-ſix.

SPRING, 1756.

March. The firſt eighteen days moſtly dry: thence to the twenty-ſixth froſt, ſnow, and hail: thence to the end cloudy and wet. Winds variable.

April. A very moiſt and cold month, frequent ſhowers, and gluts of rain and hail. Winds moſtly N.W. or ſome point of the E.

May. The fore half of the month alternately cloudy, ſhowery, and fair, and very cold: hail and ſnow at the beginning. The twelfth and thirteenth perpetual rain of near forty-eight hours continuance, wind S. E. The fifteenth a warm ſummer's day: the latter half of the month moſtly fair. Winds N. W. at the beginning; afterwards E. S. E. and N. E.

A ge-

A general healthineſs prevailed through the three ſpring months, very few fevers, and ſcarce any diſorders, except our endemics, as coughs, colds, and diſorders of the lungs, which were very frequent throughout theſe three months, with the chin-coughs mentioned laſt quarter, which continued in March ; and in May hectics and conſumptions.

Of the few feveriſh patients that occurred to my obſervation this quarter, one recovered with a critical ſweat the ſeventh day; two died in ſeven days or leſs; one recovered in fourteen days ; one in thirteen ; one died in thirteen days ; one recovered in twenty-one days.

SUMMER.

June. A wet and winter-like month for the moſt part ; few days wholly free from rain : the ſeventeenth and twenty-fourth at night great gluts of rain : towards the end warm and pleaſant. Winds S. W. ſometimes S. E. but both attended with rain.

July.

July. Excepting the firſt ſix days, which were moſtly fair, the reſt of the month was cloudy, with ſhowers interſperſed, and few intirely fair days: more rain near the end, particularly the twenty-third. The principal winds S. E. and N. E.

Auguſt. The winter-like weather continued the beginning of this month, then it was alternately cloudy, gloomy, and fair to the middle: thence to the end very frequent rains, and the ſtreets dirty, as in winter: the twenty-ſecond at night a great fall of rain. The winds variable.

A wet ſummer, but healthy; no epidemic diſeaſes; fevers rare. In the fore part of June and in July, coughs and colds were frequent. In a mountainous tract near Dublin, Baltibois, ſore mouths, affecting the gums and palate, were frequent, even in adults, and at the ſame time I ſaw in town two old perſons alike affected.

Of the fevers that occurred to my obſervation this quarter, one with a ſore

throat

throat terminated in four days, a peripneumonic fever ended in a critical ſweat the ſeventh day, though the criſis was not perfect; one the eighth day by a critical ſweat, with a ſlight relapſe; one the ninth day imperfectly by ſweat, completely the twelfth day; one peripneumonic in fifteen days, but the ſeparation in the urine not completed until the twentieth day; one in fourteen days; one miliary, the eruption appearing the fifteenth day, but his fever did not leave him till the twenty-eighth.

AUTUMN.

September. Alternately fair and gloomy, and rains frequently interſperſed: the third, fifth, fourteenth, and twenty-ſecond, much rain: the twenty-fifth, twenty-ſixth, twenty-ſeventh, on a ſudden ſultry and windy, with a heavy hygrometer. The principal winds S. E. E. and N. E.

October. Scarce a day without rain moſt of the month until the twenty-ſecond; the

the ſecond and third, ſeventh and nineteenth, gluts of rain: the ſecond at night a ſtorm; but the ſeventh in the morning early a great ſtorm, deſtructive to men and ſhipping: from the twenty-ſecond to the end, moſtly dry and pleaſant. Winds moſtly S. E.

November. Fair weather prevailed throughout the month: from the eighteenth to the twenty-fourth froſt: the ſeventeenth and twenty-ſixth rainy: the month concluded mild and ſummer-like. The principal winds N. W. and S. E.

It was a healthy autumn; few fevers attended, and thoſe I obſerved were of the low kind, v. g. one miliary, and attended with hemorrhages fatal the tenth day: another terminated happily the tenth or eleventh day: a third died the ninth.

Fluxes attended the moiſt month of October, which alſo accompanied ſome of the fevers of late, which proved fatal.

In November the meazles were very frequent, but not mortal.

WIN-

WINTER, 1756, 1757.

December. The prevailing weather was dry, and either ſerene or foggy: the fourth, the thirteenth at night, and the fifteenth, rainy: ſome days pleaſant like ſummer: it ended froſty: The principal wind S. E.

January. The froſty weather continued through the greateſt part of this month, with frequent ſnows, and ſeveral gluts of rain, particularly the ninth at night, the eighteenth at night, and the twenty-firſt and twenty-fifth. The twelfth at night a violent ſtorm at S. E. which did great damage to the ſhipping. The principal wind S. E.

February. Froſt and ſnow at the beginning: the ſixth at night a great fall of rain, fair afterwards great part of the month, though ſometimes cloudy and windy near the end. The principal winds S. W.

SUMMARY.

Spring variable, a cold and moiſt April. Sum-

Summer very wet.

Autumn variable.

Winter frosty.

The winter was healthy, except that coughs and colds attended, particularly in December, and remarkably at the latter end of it on the sudden change to cold; and during the months of January and February, coughs, inflammatory colds, sore eyes, and swelled jaws, chiefly prevailed; and the asthmatic suffered greatly, and several of them died.

Total buried this year one thousand five hundred and fifty.

SPRING, 1757.

March. A wet month; sometimes a little frost, particularly the fourth, fifth, and sixth, and frequently hail, and two notable storms the fifteenth and twenty-third, which did considerable damage. The twenty-first and twenty-fourth a great glut of rain: from the fifteenth till near the end windy. The principal winds W. and N. W.

April.

April. Variable, but with a prevalence of cold weather, and a very backward ſpring: the firſt three days wet and cold, thence to the ninth warm, thence to the end frequent rain and hail, and ſome ſnow: it concluded warm and fair. The principal wind S. W.

May. Generally dry and cool: from the eleventh to the ſixteenth ſhowery, as alſo at the end. The principal winds N. W. W. and S. W.

The cold nipping ſpring was ſenſibly felt by divers invalids, and it proved fatal to ſeveral of the aged and conſumptively diſpoſed. Colds attended all the three months, and ſome in the warm weather ſucceeding the cold, as well as in the ſerene; but ſharp weather attended, with E. winds.

Intermitting fevers, which had not appeared ſince April 1746, came on at the end of February and beginning of March, and continued in April, which with inflammatory diſorders, pleuriſies, and coughs, were the prevailing diſeaſes in the laſt named month.

In

In May colds, rheumatifms, inflammatory fevers, and intermittents, were the principal difeafes.

SUMMER.

June. Generally fair, dry, and warm, and the principal winds N. E. S. E. or E. The fecond at night rain, as alfo the feventeenth, nineteenth, and twentieth day, and the twenty-fecond at night.

July. Somewhat cloudy at the beginning: from the feventh to the thirteenth ferene and hot, and the winds for the moft part E. The heat lefs after the thunder the fourteenth, thence to the end frequent and plentiful rains, and the winds S. W. W. and S.

Auguft. Except the feventh and eighth, which were fair and hot, there were few days but cloudy or wet, or both: and the latter end was fqually, cold, and winter-like. The principal winds N. W. S. W. and W.

During the three fummer-months the pre-

prevailing fevers were evidently of the putrid and petechial kind, and ſometimes attended with miliary puſtules. There was a gangrenous tendency in ſome of their ſores by bliſters and otherwiſe. The attack was frequently mild and deceitful.

One died the tenth, another the fourteenth day, two recovered the fourteenth or fifteenth day : with three the fever ran out to the nineteenth, twenty-firſt, and twenty-ſecond.

In June and the beginning of July, ſeveral cutaneous diſorders appeared, probably owing to the extraordinary heat of the weather, which attended ſome part of thoſe months; and in both thoſe months I met with ſome dyſenteries among the poor, promoted, perhaps, by the badneſs of their bread, as it was a time of great ſcarcity.

AUTUMN.

September. Excepting the two firſt days, the weather was generally fair and dry,

dry, or gloomy and pleaſant, with a prevalence of S. E. and N. E. winds.

October. The dry weather continued through the greateſt part of this month, ſo that there was very little rain, except on the fifth at night, with a ſtorm, and on the ſeventh at night; but ſeveral ſummer-like days, and a few fogs and ſlight froſts, at the latter end. The principal winds N. W. S. W. and W.

November. After a ſeries of nearly two months dry weather, ſucceeded a winter-like ſeaſon of frequent rain and wind throughout the month, after the fourth day. On the tenth dreadful thunder and lightning: the fifteenth and nineteenth ſtormy. The principal wind S. W.

In autumn the prevailing fevers were ſtill of the low and putrid kind, attended with a weak and quick pulſe, though ſometimes ſcarcely quick, and even ſlower than in health. Petechial and ſometimes miliary eruptions appeared at uncertain times, and tremors; and as the diſeaſe advanced,

advanced, a delirium or ſome degree of it, and a coma. A bilious diarrhœa uſually attended, and ſeemed to be ſalutary.

The time of the criſis was various, moſt frequently on the fourteenth day, though to ſome it proved fatal ſooner, and more rarely ran out to the twenty-firſt.

At the cloſe of October this fever became more frequent, and often proved fatal, as it did likewiſe in November to not a few of the young and ſtrong; and we received accounts of a like malignity attending this fever in the country.

Bliſters in the advanced ſtate of the fever were of ſervice, though not always ſucceſsful. The ſmall-pox ſeemed to keep pace with the fever in reſpect to malignity.

WINTER, 1757, 1758.

December. Moiſt the firſt ſix days, then gloomy, foggy, and cloudy, with frequent ſlight froſts, and ſometimes a heavy hygrometer, with a high barometer:

ter: pleaſant for the ſeaſon: the fourth perpetual rain, the twenty-ninth a ſummer-like day. The principal winds N. W.

January. A dry month: after a little ſnow at the beginning, the firſt fifteen days were mild, and alternately ſerene and cloudy, ſometimes a little wet; thence to the twenty-fourth froſt, and a little ſnow; thence to the end gloomy and pleaſant for the ſeaſon. The principal winds S. E. and S. W.

February. The pleaſant weather continued the firſt ſix days, which was ſucceeded by frequent rains, and winds; ſome ſnow and froſt through the reſt of the month: the eighth and twelfth ſtormy: the nineteenth a great fall of ſnow. The principal winds W. and S. W.

SUMMARY.

Spring cold and backward.

Summer generally cloudy and wet, except June, and a few days in July and Auguſt.

Autumn

Autumn moſtly dry and ſummer-like.

Winter moſtly mild and open.

The predominant diſeaſes throughout the winter-quarter are ſaid to have been of the inflammatory kind, as pleuriſies, coughs, colds, ſore throats, and obſtinate inflammations of the eyes in February, in which month the inflammatory fevers are ſaid to have partaken of the low petechial kind: but the principal fevers that occurred to my obſervation in the winter-quarter, were of the low petechial kind; and in January that article was increaſed much beyond the uſual number, where alſo it is obſervable that the ſmall-pox kept pace in malignity with the fevers. The diarrhœa that attended proved ſalutary, as laſt autumn.

The time of the criſis was various, as the eleventh, twelfth, fourteenth, ſixteenth, and twenty-firſt days.

Bliſters were ſtill of ſervice in the advanced ſtate of the fever, notwithſtanding the putrid diſpoſition of the juices.

Total buried this year one thouſand eight hundred and twenty-five; or, according

ing to a calculation perhaps more accurate, one thoufand fix hundred and thirty-nine.

SPRING, 1758.

March. Variable, moftly cold, and a backward fpring: frequent rain, and fometimes fnow: it concluded fair, pleafant, and warm. The principal winds S. E. N. E. and E.

April. Serene and cold, rain and fhowers interfperfed, and thefe frequently of hail or fnow: the twelfth, the fixteenth in the night, and the twentieth, plenty of rain. It ended fair and dry. The principal winds E. S. E. and N. W.

May. Moftly fair and dry; fcarce any rain, except the great glut on the thirtieth, with thunder: from the eighteenth to near the end, very warm: it ended cool. The principal winds S. E. E. and N. E.

The petechial fevers lately prevailing did not wholly ceafe in this city, nor in feveral of the north and weft parts of the kingdom during the months of March and April; and thofe that fell under my ob-

ferſervation in the laſt month proved fatal the eighth, fourteenth, and ſixteenth days; and it was obſervable that many fevers which attacked with inflammatory ſymptoms, did not bear bleeding.

Pleuriſies, peripneumonies, and rheumatiſms, were very frequent in March: alſo in this month and the beginning of April a fever was frequent, which ſeized chiefly young girls, and terminated in a few days with eryſipelatous eruptions all over the ſkin.

The month of May was as remarkable for better health as for good weather; nevertheleſs, during the three months, but eſpecially April and May, our endemial diſeaſes, coughs and colds, were frequent, and thoſe of bad lungs ſuffered much; alſo ſome pleuriſies attended, in two of which the criſis ſucceeded happily by ſweat, as very frequently happens; in one the ſixth, in the other the eighth day.

SUM-

SUMMER.

June. Fair and dry moftly, fo that the feventh and fixteenth were the only days remarkable for rain: it was alfo frequently cold, and fome days winter-like; but the twenty-fifth and twenty-fixth very hot. The principal winds W. N. W. and S. W.

July. Generally cloudy and wet; not many days free from rain: the fourteenth a glut of rain: fome very few hot and fultry days, but more cool and winter-like. The principal winds N. W.

Auguft. Frequently fultry, gloomy, and fair alternately, and likewife often rainy, efpecially in and near Dublin, where we had plentiful rains. The principal winds S. W. and N. W. It concluded fair and cool, with northerly winds.

About the beginning of June there was a fudden change of the weather to cold, which was attended with coughs, chin-coughs, fore throats, quinzies, pleurifies, peripneumonies, and rheumatifms, moft of

which

which diſorders continued during great part of the remainder of the wet ſummer, viz. in July and the beginning of Auguſt.

In June the fevers ſeemed to border on the intermittent kind, having a notable exacerbation, with chillineſs in the evening.

July was attended with inflammatory fevers, and likewiſe with thoſe of the low petechial kind, in divers caſes of which the time of the criſis was various; as on the ſixth, fourteenth, twentieth, and twenty-eighth days. Dyſenteries alſo were frequent in July, ſome of which were obſtinate.

In Auguſt the cholera morbus occurred, and dyſenteries continued to be frequent; and the ſmall-pox, which had been mild and diſtinct before, became very frequent, and were of a confluent and bad kind.

AUTUMN.

September. A fine harveſt month, moſtly dry, pleaſant, and cool; ſome little froſts, and the principal wind N. W. The ſecond

ſecond at night rainy: the ſeventeenth a great fall of rain: the ſixth ſtormy.

October. The dry weather continued to the twentieth, except the ſeventh and eighth days, which were wet: in the latter part of the period mentioned were frequent froſts: from the twentieth to the end cloudy, wet, and ſometimes windy: the twenty-ſeventh at night a ſtorm, and much rain. The principal winds S. E. E. and N. W.

November. Frequent rains throughout the month: a good deal the twentieth. Windy the fourteenth, ſeventeenth, eighteenth, and nineteenth; elſe cloudy, and ſome little fogs: not long fair. The principal wind S. W.

The autumn in general was healthy, and the fevers not generally malignant, but rather ſlight and favourable; and during the three months, the inflammatory fevers to thoſe of the putrid kind, was near double or treble of the firſt to the laſt; and the putrid ſort generally terminated in nine or fifteen days, and ſeveral of theſe had diarrhœas through the whole courſe of the fever.

The meazles were frequent, and often of a bad kind during the three months: and the chin-cough was frequent in September and November.

A ſudden onſet of cold towards the end of September introduced epidemic colds, which, beſide ſome ſore throats, prevailed both in town and country, and continued through October.

Beſides the meazles, there were alſo pretty frequent in October and November certain eruptive fevers among children, and attended with the like cough and difficulty of breathing as the meazles, which did not ſeem to require a different method of cure; and November exhibited ſome ſcarlet fevers.

WINTER, 1758, 1759.

December. A froſt and ſome ſnow from the fifth to the ſeventh. Windy from the eighth to the ſixteenth: elſe for the moſt part rainy; and gluts of rain the eleventh,

venth, ſeventeenth, twentieth, and twenty-ty-ſixth at nights. The principal wind S. W.

January. Very windy to the ſeventeenth, and ſhowers interſperſed, and ſometimes blew a ſtorm, particularly the ſeventh, ninth, and thirteenth, and commonly blew chiefly in the evenings and nights: a warm month like ſpring; ſome fogs after the ſtormy weather, but without froſt. The principal winds S. W. and W.

February. A fine dry month for the moſt part, and a good deal of it like ſummer: windy the fifth. A little froſt about the ſixteenth, ſeventeenth, and eighteenth. The twenty-fifth and twenty-ſixth much rain, with wind S. E. The principal winds S. W. and S. E.

SUMMARY.

Spring cold and dry.
Summer rainy for the moſt part.
Autumn moſtly dry and fair.
Winter mild.

The diſeaſes in December and January were chiefly of the inflammatory kind; as fevers,

fevers, attended with violent coughs, pleurisies, pains of the breaſt, and ſome hæmoptoes. The few fevers that occurred to my obſervation, in December, were ſlight and favourable, in two of which the criſis fell on the fifth and ſeventh days, being by ſweat; in a third, being by a diarrhœa, it was protracted to the fourteenth. The meazles did not wholly diſappear in December; and ſome children of weakly conſtitutions ſuffered much by them, their lungs and bowels being left in a vitiated ſtate.

In January, beſides the meazles, the ſcarlet fever, which had infeſted the autumn, ſtill continued.

February was remarkable for great health as well as fine weather: in the Infirmary the diſeaſes which prevailed moſt were ſtill of the inflammatory kind; and towards the end of the month ſome agues appeared.

A

A

SUMMARY REVIEW

OF THE

DISEASES above-mentioned, during a Series of above THIRTY YEARS, chiefly with regard to the SEASONS in which they prevailed.

1ſt. INflammatory diſeaſes in general are mentioned in the ſpring of the years 1723, 41, 43, 47, 57.

In winter 1739, 57.

Hence, and from the ſubſequent obſervations on inflammations of particular parts, ariſes a confirmation of what has been advanced by others, that the ſpring ſeaſon promotes ſuch diſeaſes, and of the criſping, coagulating quality of the N. and E. winds prevailing in that ſeaſon.

2dly. Tumours of the face, jaws, parotids, and ſore eyes, occur.

In ſpring 1739, 40, 43, 44, 45, 46, 47, 51, 53, 57.

In ſummer 1745, 48 (June and July 1756 wet).

In autumn 1737, 39.

In winter 1737, 51, 55, 56, 57.

Cor. Theſe diſorders abound moſt in ſpring, next in winter, leaſt in ſummer and autumn, when the perſpiration is freer.

3dly. Pleuriſies occur.

In ſpring 1727, 40, 44, 47, 48, 50, 57, 58.

In ſummer 1748, 58.

In autumn 1749, 58.

In winter 1739, 46, 57, 58.

4thly. Peripneumonies occur.

In ſpring 1732, 40, 44, 47, 58.

In ſummer 1758, upon a ſudden onſet of cold.

In autumn oo.

In winter 1739, 58.

Cor. Pleuriſies and peripneumonies are much more frequent in ſpring than in any other ſeaſon, and next in winter.

5thly. Sore throats occur.

In

In ſpring 1733, 35, 40, 43, 44, 45, 52, 53.

In ſummer 1735 cold and wet, 45 alſo wet, and 58 wet.

In autumn 1738, 48, 58.

In winter 1737, 39, 43, 46, 51, 57.

Cor. Sore throats are moſt frequent in ſpring, next in winter, in ſummer ſeem promoted by wet and cold weather then happening.

6thly. Coughs occur.

In ſpring 1732, 34, 45, 47, 48, 49, 51, 52, 53, 54, 55, 56, 57, 58.

In ſummer 1745, a wet one; 50, in Auguſt cold, winter-like; 53, June wet and cold. 56, June and July very wet and cold; 58, rainy.

In autumn 1746, 49, 51, 52, 53, 54, 55.

In winter 1739, 45, 46, 48, 49, 50, 51, 52, 53, 54, 55, 56, 57, 58..

1. Coughs occur in ſpring as much as in winter, and particularly in May, from the nature of the prevailing winds and weather

weather peculiar to the ſeaſon elſewhere deſcribed, which may furniſh uſeful precaution to the conſumptively diſpoſed.

2. Coughs, properly a winter and ſpring diſeaſe, infeſt the ſummers alſo when cold and wet.

To this I ſhall annex, by way of confirmation, the accounts of colds or catarrhs, which in the foregoing hiſtory occur.

In ſpring 1736, 39, 41, 42, 43, 44, 47, 49, 50, 53, 55, 56, 57, 58.

In ſummer 48, 53, 56 (of theſe three two were wet.)

In autumn 1729, 38, 39, 47, 50, 51, 53, 55, 58.

In winter 1736, 37, 39, 43, 44, 47, 54, 56.

Here, the ſpring is conſiderably more productive of colds and catarrhs than winter; and the autumn as much as winter, from the ſudden changes to cold then frequently happening.

And

And the epidemic far-ſpreading catarrhs and catarrhal fevers, noticed in the above hiſtory, made their appearance chiefly in autumn and winter, particularly that in November 1729, common to us and England at the ſame time, attended with a ſlight fever; another in winter 1736, which was alſo common to us and England at the ſame time; and that in autumn 1758, and the catarrhal fever in winter 1732; that in October 1737, and a third of the ſame kind called the influenza in ſpring 1743: but it is obſervable, that in this laſt ſeaſon, it was the moſt favourable, or leaſt mortal. See the obſervations in 1743.

7thly. Conſumptions occur.

In ſpring 1750, 51, 53, 54, 55, 56, 57.

In ſummer and autumn oo.

In winter 1753, 56, viz. more in ſpring than in any other ſeaſon.

8thly. Intermitting fevers occur.

In ſpring 1725, 28, 29, 30, 32, 33, 34,

34, 35, 36, 38, 39, 44, 45, 48, 49, 50, 51, 52, 53, 54, 57.

In ſummer 1728; 33, partly wet; 34, 35, wet ſeaſons; 36, hot; 38, cold and wet; 45, 49, both wet; 50, June and Auguſt, cold and winter-like.

1751, A wet ſummer; 58, rainy.

In autumn 1732, 33, 36.

In winter 1732, 34, 49, 50, 57, 58.

COR. Intermitting fevers are properly a ſpring-diſeaſe, but ſometimes, eſpecially in moiſt and cold ſeaſons, become a ſummer one, as is before obſerved of coughs; elſe much more rare in any other ſeaſon than in ſpring, the ſeaſon of the N. and E. winds, which I apprehend may deſerve to be conſidered.

9thly. The putrid, petechial, and low nervous fever occurred.

In ſpring 1729, 40, 41, 50, 57, 58.

In ſummer 1725, and not mortal; 29, 32; ſporadic, July 35; 36, 40, 41; 45, all the year ſporadically, and in an otherwiſe healthy ſeaſon, and wet ſummer; 47, hot and dry; Auguſt 51, in an other-

wiſe

wiſe healthy ſeaſon, but a wet ſummer; 55, wet and cold; 57, cloudy and wet; July 58, rainy.

Autumn 1725, not mortal; 29, 32, 33, 34, 40, 54, 55, 56, alſo healthy; 57, 58.

Winter 1728, 34; 35, mortal; 37; 46, moſt mortal in winter; 48, 54, ſporadic; 55, 57.

Cor. The low and putrid fever is very frequent with us, and ſeems to be proper to our climate; for in the compaſs of theſe obſervations, few years, perhaps none, were wholly exempt from it: it has been obſerved to attend in ſeaſons otherwiſe healthy, and in all ſeaſons of the year, though leaſt in ſpring; and where it has been truly petechial, it has ſometimes proved benign, not malignant, though too often otherwiſe; and the obſervations of our late Engliſh writers, that this fever attends moſtly in or after moiſt ſeaſons, ſeem to hold here alſo.

As a confirmation of the truth of the above obſervations, I ſhall here ſubjoin an eſtimate, at a medium, of the numbers dying

dying in each quarter refpectively of fome of the moft remarkable of the difeafes above fpecified, made by an eminent phyfician, the late Dr. Bryan Robinfon, for near the fpace of forty years preceding the commencement of my obfervations, and which may ferve as a reciprocal confirmation of the truth of each.

"1. The greateft number of deaths from fever was in the winter-quarter, and next in fummer; in the firft, eighteen thoufand two hundred and eighty; in the laft, as feventeen thoufand five hundred twenty-three, though the fummer number was alfo greater than that of fpring or fall *.

"2. Of intermitting fevers, the far greater number died in the fpring-quarter.

"3. Of the pleurify, the greateft number in the fpring-quarter, and next in the winter-quarter.

"4. Of the fmall-pox, the greateft number died in the fummer and autumnal quarter.

* During a feries of twenty-eight years fucceeding; alfo the greateft number of deaths from fever, was in the winter-quarter, though the leaft in fummer.

Of

" 5. Of the conſumption, the greateſt number in winter, next in ſpring."

I ſhall next, from the diaries I kept, give the time of the criſis or termination of fevers, whether putrid, inflammatory, or mixed, as far as noted down in the preceding hiſtory, collected in a great meaſure from obſervations on the poor, where few medicines were uſed, and ſo nature was leaſt diſguiſed.

1. The days on which the putrid and low fevers in the preceding hiſtory terminated were, as in the two following tables.

TABLE I.

Days of the termination of the putrid and low fevers	5	6	7	9	10	11	16	19	20	21	22	23	24	28	42
N° of patients	1	2	1	2	3	4	2	2	2	7	1	1	1	2	1

Thus it appears that the moſt frequent period of the putrid low fever was nearly three weeks, or a day or two over or under the twenty firſt day.

TABLE

TABLE II.

Days of the termination of the inflammatory and mixed fevers.	1	2	4	5	6	7	8	9	13	14	15	17	19	20	21	23
Nº. of patients.	1	1	2	9	6	9	3	4	2	8	1	3	1	1	2	1

Hence it appears that the fifth, ſeventh, and fourteenth days nearly, were the moſt frequent periods of the inflammatory and mixed fevers.

See a farther illuſtration of this matter in the ſubſequent review of the following ſeven years.

To theſe two tables, drawn from obſervation in Dublin, it may not be improper to add a third, expreſſing alſo the number of the patients, and the ſeveral days that proved critical, either in their recovery or death, from Hippocrates's Epidemics, in which appears a far greater affinity between their fevers and ours with reſpect to the term of the duration of each than might be imagined; and at the ſame time by this account compared with

with the modern accounts given of the periods of their fevers in the Eaſt Indies, Egypt, and in the warmer countries in America, that in theſe hotter countries their fevers are more rapid, and finiſh their courſe much ſooner than thoſe deſcribed by Galen and Hippocrates; whereas ours, in a cooler climate, are leſs violent, ſlower, and of longer duration than either.

Of thoſe in the epidemics, the following is a ſketch:

In 2 days 2,	In 80 days 2,	In 8 days 3,	In 40 days 6,
In 3 days 7,	In 4 days 7,	In 17 days 7,	In 9 days 10,
In 11 days 11,	In 6 days 12,	In 5 days 14,	In 14 days 18,
In 20, 21, and 23 days 20,		In 7 days 28.	

So that in thoſe epidemics the greateſt number finiſhed their courſe in ſeven days, the next in three weeks nearly, the next in fourteen days, &c.

COROL-

COROLLARIES.

1. Notwithſtanding the variableneſs of our climate, not admitting of ſuch ſtated periods in the return of diſeaſes as in the warmer countries, where their winds and weather are in a great meaſure fixed and regular; yet, even here, we plainly trace ſomething of a periodical revolution, particularly in the above ſummary review of the ſeaſons of the year proper to inflammations of the face and jaws, anginas, pleuriſies, peripnumonies, coughs, and catarrhs.

2. The time of the criſis of fevers, whether putrid or inflammatory, is very uncertain and various; and yet the ſeventh and fourteenth days, or nearly ſo, appear to be the days in which the greateſt number of our inflammatory fevers terminate, as the twenty-firſt is nearly that in which the low and putrid fevers end, as in Hypocrates's Epidemics; and it is worthy of obſervation, that this is the longeſt term which

which Hypocrates aſſigns to diſeaſes properly denominated acute *. And I have frequently obſerved where they have ended much ſooner, v. g. in five days, the patients have been liable to relapſes, as though the depuration were not ordinarily completed in ſo ſhort a time.

To this account agrees Fernelius's obſervation in France: " Continuam febrem ſecunda, aut (quod tardiſſimum eſt) tertia hebdomada decretorie ſolvit. Si qua continua febris ſupra 21um. diem exporrigatur, hanc tu ſymptomaticam cenſeto, atque eam vel interiore phlegmone aut abſceſſu, vel ex putredine viſceri alicui impacta profectam."

3. The putrid and low fevers are ſlower in their progreſs, and of longer duration, than the inflammatory. Of the firſt the inſtances of a termination in five or ſix days are rare, of the laſt very frequent: the firſt very frequently ran out to three weeks, the laſt rarely: the firſt have con-

* Le Clerc Hiſtoire de la Medecine.

tinued

tinued ſix weeks, the laſt never in the above hiſtory.

But to proceed :

10thly. Diarrhœas occurred.

In ſpring 00.

In ſummer 1731.

In autumn 1731, 33, 35, 36, 56.

In winter 1733.

11thly. Dyſenteries occurred.

In ſpring 41, 49, 57.

In ſummer 1737, 40, 57, 58.

In autumn 1733, 36, 37, 39, 40, 52, 54, 58.

In winter 1733, 44, 52, 54, 58.

12thly. The cholera morbus occurred.

In ſpring 00.

In ſummer, July 1726, June and Auguſt 57, Auguſt 58.

In Autumn, September, and October, 1736, 50.

13thly. Of the ſmall-pox.

The chief thing that ſeems worthy of notice is, that beſides their raging in hot weather, Huxham's obſervation is confirmed,

firmed, that, as in the petechial and putrid fevers, they frequently prove of a bad kind in and after wet ſeaſons, as in the ſummer of 1738, of 45, 52, and Auguſt 58.

In order to a further illuſtration of this matter, I ſhall now ſum up from a ſynoptic table which I drew from the preceding hiſtory of the ſeaſons and diſeaſes, the reſpective numbers of the times in the ſeveral ſeaſons, in which ſome of the moſt notable of our prevailing diſeaſes were obſerved, which, as far as the evidence afforded by thoſe obſervations made in Dublin for thirty-ſix years, viz. from 1725 to 1761 incluſive, can be allowed, may furniſh ſome concluſions of uſe and importance; concluſions drawn not by idle and random gueſſes, but by fair induction from facts, minuted down, and faithfully related, with a ſole view to the diſcovery of truth.

We find then in the foregoing hiſtory, and the continuation of it to the year 1761 incluſive,

1ſt.

1ſt. That agues or intermittent fevers were obſerved,

In ſpring	19	times.
Summer	4	
Autumn	1	
Winter	0	

2dly. Coughs, colds, and catarrhs were obſerved,

In ſpring	24	times.
Summer	6	
Autumn	11	
Winter	18	

Chin-coughs were obſerved,

In ſpring	3	times.
Summer	1	
Autumn	2	
Winter	1	

3dly. Tumors, inflammations, and excoriations, affecting the face, eyes, ears, mouth, and jaws, were obſerved,

In ſpring	11	times.
Summer	00	
Autumn	2	
Winter	5	

From

From all which, it abundantly appears, that the ſpring-ſeaſon, more than any other, is attended by coughs and defluxions, even more than the winter; and undoubtedly the N. and E. winds, uſually then predominant, have a principal ſhare in this.

It alſo appears that intermittent fevers are a true vernal diſeaſe, even according to the poet,

> Each ſeaſon doth its poiſon bring,
> Rheums chill the winter, agues blaſt the ſpring.

But this wants a comment; for aſſuredly, according to what has been obſerved in Dublin during the period above-mentioned, the ſpring is conſiderably more productive of defluxions than the winter; and therefore the firſt comes rather *nigro carbone notanda* to invalids than winter, whoſe blaſts are generally tempered from the weſt and ſouth.

Agreeable to this are the following obſervations concerning ſore throats, pleuriſies,

risies, and the meazles, from which the cough is inseparable, viz.

4thly. Sore throats and quinsies in the above synopsis were observed,

In spring	7	times.
Summer	4	
Autumn	1	
Winter	5	

5thly. Pleurisies and peripneumonies,

In spring	8	times.
Summer	1	
Autumn	1	
Winter	5	

6thly. The meazles,

In spring	4	times.
Summer	00	
Autumn	2	
Winter	1	

7thly. Fevers inflammatory,

In spring	3	times.
Summer	1	
Autumn	1	
Winter	3	

8thly.

8thly. Fevers low, nervous, putrid, petechial, and miliary,

In ſpring	5	times.
Summer	8	
Autumn	12	
Winter	9	

9thly. Diarrhœas occur,

In ſpring	1	times.
Summer	00	
Autumn	9	
Winter	5	

COR. The diarrhœa is plainly an autumnal diſeaſe.

10thly. Dyſenteries,

In ſpring	2	times.
Summer	5	
Autumn	10	
Winter	4	

COR. The dyſentery is alſo an autumnal diſeaſe.

11th. The cholera morbus is noted,

In

In ſpring	00	times.
Summer	2	
Autumn	3	
Winter	00	

And to conclude, I ſhall here ſubjoin a compariſon of the epidemic diſeaſes of Dublin and Paris with regard to the ſeaſons, from obſervations publiſhed in the Memoirs of the Royal Academy, from the year 1746 to 1752; from whence it will appear, that notwithſtanding the difference of the climate in both places, there is a greater ſimilarity in the prevailing diſeaſes, and a more conſtant connexion between theſe and the ſeaſons, than might be imagined: for it appears, from a like ſummary review of the obſervations mentioned made in Paris,

1. That pleuriſies, peripneumonies, and inflammations of the breaſt, occur moſt in winter and ſpring, not in ſummer, more rarely in autumn.

2. Catarrhs, colds, and coughs, occur in both places in all ſeaſons, but leaſt in ſummer;

mer; though even in this ſeaſon, when it proves very moiſt, a ſudden change to cold commonly introduces them: and in the French regiſtry they are much more prevalent in moiſt, than in dry ſeaſons; the watry vapours in moiſt fogs, and otherwiſe, being more plentifully imbibed by the venæ bibulæ, diſperſed over the external and internal ſurface of the body.

3. The Pariſian and Dublin regiſtries agree in making intermittent fevers to be a ſpring-diſeaſe; for at Paris, as well as here, they are comparatively rare in winter, but become frequent through the ſpring-months. In Paris alſo they are rare in ſummer until Auguſt, and continue frequent through autumn; and it is obſervable, that their intermittents were much more frequently attended with fair and dry weather than with exceſſive moiſture.

4. Putrid or malignant fevers occur in moſt months of the year in the French regiſtry, as well as ours; but it is obſervable, that the fevers that paſs under this de-

denomination in theirs, occur more in dry than in moiſt weather.

5. Their catarrhous fevers were moſtly attended with moiſture.

6. Dyſenteries in the French regiſtry ſcarce appear in ſpring or ſummer; but infeſt chiefly the autumnal months, or at leaſt from Auguſt to November incluſive: and moreover it is obſervable in the French regiſtry, as well as by ſome late obſervations in Dublin, that this diſeaſe is much more frequently accompanied by hot and dry than moiſt weather; a probable argument that it is not ſo much owing to a ſtoppage of perſpiration as to inflammation and an exaltation of the juices to a more acrid ſtate in hot and dry weather, although the autumnal ſeaſon advancing, and attended with a decreaſe in the perſpiration, muſt undoubtedly determine the humours more to the bowels: and to this the two following obſervations ſeems to agree, viz.

7. Diarrhœas prevail chiefly in the autumnal months in both regiſtries, from Auguſt

Auguſt to November incluſive; are leſs frequent in winter; rare in ſpring and ſummer, as is obſerved above concerning dyſenteries, diarrhœas; alſo in the French regiſtry are much more frequently attended with hot and dry weather than an exceſs of moiſture.

8. In the French regiſtry ſcarce any inſtance occurs of an epidemic cholic in winter or ſpring, but in ſummer and the beginning of autumn; chiefly in Auguſt and September, in hot and dry weather.

Theſe laſt obſervations agree with thoſe made in a different climate, even thoſe of the divine old man in his books de Morbis Epidemicis, viz. "Cholericæ affectiones magis æſtate fiunt: æſtate & autumno lienteriæ, dyſenteriæ, teneſmi & alvi profluvia."

HIS-

HISTORY

OF THE

WEATHER

AND

DISEASES in DUBLIN.

N.B. The reader is desired to remember in making any comparisons between the observations before and since the commencement of the New Stile, which was introduced with the year 1752, that each month since this year takes in eleven days of the subsequent month, according to the Old Stile, obtaining before the year 1752.

H I S T O R Y

OF THE

W E A T H E R

AND

DISEASES in DUBLIN, for SEVEN YEARS, continued.

S P R I N G, 1759.

IN March the weather was variable as uſual: the principal winds W. and N.W.

Winds.	March.
N. E.	2
E.	2
S. E.	2
N.	3
S. W.	3
N. W.	12
W.	12

April was moſtly fair and dry, ending ſerene and cold. The principal winds N. W. and ſome point of the E. as E. and N. E.

	April.
S. E.	5
N.	3
E.	7
N. E.	8
N. W.	10
S.	1
S. W.	1
W.	5

May

May.		
S. E.	4	May was for the moſt part fair and dry: frequently ſharp in the mornings and evenings, and ſome froſts: near the end hot, concluded very cold. The principal winds N. E. N. W. and S. W.
N.	5	
N. E.	9	
W.	6	
N. W.	7	
S. W.	8	

The chief diſeaſes in the ſpring months were colds and catarrhs in divers ſhapes, coughs, and aſthmas; and ſeveral tabid perſons were carried off in April.

In May, among other diſorders of the breaſt, there were ſome pleuriſies; in one of which was an imperfect criſis by ſweat the fifth or ſixth day.

At the king's infirmary, inflammatory fevers during theſe ſpring-months to the ſlow putrid kind, were nearly as fifty of the firſt to ten of the laſt.

SUMMER.

June.		
N. W.	10	Excepting the firſt half of June, the three ſummer months
S. W.	8	

were

were generally fair, dry, and warm, and ſometimes very hot; ſo that it was one of the warmeſt and drieſt ſummers, the thermometer half a degree higher than in 1757, which was a remarkably hot ſummer.

W.	7
S.	2
S. E.	7
N.	3
E.	1

In June the principal winds were N. W. and S. W.

In July N. W. and S. E.

July.	
N. W.	11
S. E.	11
S. W.	8
W.	5
N.	2
S.	1
E.	1

In Auguſt W. S. W. and N. W.

Auguſt.	
W.	12
S. W.	10
N. W.	8
E.	5
S. E.	3
N. E.	3

In June ſome dyſenteries began to make their appearance, and in July they became much more frequent, eſpecially among

young

young children, as alſo other diſorders of the ſtomach and bowels; and in Auguſt dyſenteries proceeded to ſpread among both young and old, which for the moſt part proved tractable, though in ſome few fatal, probably through want of proper advice.

Several ſevere colds attended in July, and ſome in Auguſt.

In the king's infirmary in the three ſummer-months, were about thitry-eight of the inflammatory fevers to ſix putrid.

Of the acute fevers that occurred during theſe three ſummer-months, the greater part terminated the ſeventh day by a critical ſweat, ſome the eighth, one the ninth day, one the ſixth day with ſalivation, one the fourth day with ſuppurating puſtules on the lips.

It is worthy remark, that as this ſummer, like thoſe of 1740, 1741, had been one of the warmeſt and drieſt, ſo it was likewiſe fertile in dyſenteries: but there was this difference in the two ſeaſons, that the preſent

preſent was a very plentiful one, abounding with wholeſome proviſions; whereas, in the other, proviſions were very ſcarce and bad, which no doubt muſt have increaſed the malignity of the diſeaſe.

AUTUMN.

September was generally fair, with excellent harveſt-weather. The principal winds W. S. E. and E.

September.	
W.	9
S. E.	8
E.	8
N. W.	4
S. W.	4
S.	2
N.	1
N. E.	1

October was partly fair, and ſometimes hot, like ſummer; elſe variable, with ſome gluts of rain. The principal winds W. and S. W.

October.	
W.	11
S. W.	10
S. E.	6
N. W.	4
N. E.	4
S.	3
N.	2
E.	1

November was moderate and mild, alternately gloomy and fair, with ſome froſts. The principal wind W.

November.	
W.	11
N. W.	7
S. E.	5
S.	3
S. W.	3
N.	3
N. E.	2

In

In September a few inflammatory and pleuritic fevers appeared: the ſymptoms were generally mild, and ſeveral of them terminated happily by a critical ſweat within the ſeventh day. The dyſentery was the prevailing diſeaſe, not only of this month, but of the whole quarter; and diarrhœas were not unfrequent: divers feveriſh and other diſorders were obſerved to attack the bowels.

Diarrhœas and dyſenteries continued through the months of October and November; and the laſt named diſeaſe attacked ſome of all ages.

WINTER, 1759, 1760.

December.	
W.	4
N.W.	3
N.	1
N.E.	6
E.	4
S.E.	9
S.	1
S.W.	3

December was in general cloudy and gloomy: a few fair days, ſome froſts, but more moiſt fogs. The twenty-fifth at night a ſtorm. The principal winds S. E. and N. E.

In

In January were frequent rains, ſome floods, ſleet, and ſnow. The principal winds S.W. W. S.E. and N.E.

January.	
W.	5
N.W.	4
S.E.	5
N.E.	5
E.	5
S.	1
S.W.	7

February was extremely variable, frequent and plentiful rains and floods; ſome froſts and fogs; a great fall of ſnow the fifteenth; ſeveral fair days; often windy; it ended fair, calm, and mild. The principal winds W. S.W. and N.W.

February.	
W.	10
S.W.	9
E.	1
N.W.	10
S.E.	4
N.E.	2

The dyſentery, which infeſted the autumn, was evidently on the decline, and eaſily curable. The reigning diſeaſes during the three winter-months were coughs, catarrhs, diſorders of the cheſt, and ſome rheumatiſms.

No great number of acute fevers occurred, and thoſe moſtly benign: among which, one pleuritic, who was bled and re-

covered

covered by a critical ſweat the ſixth day, one peripneumonic, who with ſome difficulty recovered the ſeventeenth day; and three other acute fevers terminated by a critical ſweat the eighth; in one of which three there was a relapſe, but a ſecond ſweat perfected the criſis.

Yearly bill of burials in Dublin one thouſand ſeven hundred and fifty-two.

SUMMARY.

The ſpring moſtly fair and dry.

The ſummer moſtly fair, dry, and warm.

The autumn moſtly fair and moderate.

The winter variable, but more inclined to moiſture.

SPRING, 1760.

March.	
S. W.	3
N. W.	11
S. E.	4
N.	3
W.	5
S.	2
E.	4

March was uncommonly fair, dry, and duſty, and in a great meaſure free from rain and wind: ſometimes like ſummer: a few froſty mornings in the country.

country. The principal wind N. W.

April was alſo moſtly fair and dry. The principal winds from ſome point of the E. particularly the N. E. which was as frequent as the W. and S. W. It ended cold and ſharp.

April.	
E.	4
S. W.	8
W.	8
S. E.	3
N. E.	8
N. W.	2
S.	2

May was variable as to heat, cold, and ſerenity; ſometimes warm, then ſuddenly cold. The principal winds S. E. N. E. and E.

May.	
N. E.	7
S. E.	10
E.	5
W.	4
S. W.	7
N. W.	4
N.	1
S.	2

Our endemial diſeaſes, colds, coughs, aſthmas, and conſumptive diſorders prevailed greatly, ſo that I ſcarce ever obſerved a greater frequency of colds and conſumptive caſes than laſt winter, and throughout the three ſpring-months; and ſore eyes particularly attended the N. E. winds in April.

From

From hence I apprehended a conſiderable connexion between the late epidemic diſeaſe among horſes and thoſe among men; in order to illuſtrate which I have ſubjoined a ſhort hiſtory of that diſorder among the horſes, together with a review of the like diſorder among them for a ſeries of years paſt, with a compariſon of it with the epidemics prevailing among men at the ſame time.

The fevers that fell under my obſervation in May were of the acute kind, proving critical about the tenth day, and ſome on the ſixth and eighth. The ſubjects were moſtly poor, and eſcaped with very little aſſiſtance from art.

SUMMER.

June.	
S. W.	6
E.	5
S. E.	8
S.	2
W.	4
N. E.	5
N. W.	8
N.	2

June, in general, was variable, ·ather inclined to cold, v. g. the fore part of June was moſtly fair, with ſome hot days; and the winds S. E. E. and N. E. the reſt of the month moſtly

we

wet and winter-like, and the winds W. and N. W.

July was generally fair and dry, more rarely cloudy, and a little rain: a few hot days. The principal winds N. W. W. and E.

July.	
N. W	11
N. E.	3
W.	9
N.	4
S.	1
E.	5
S. E.	3
S. W.	4

In Auguſt the three firſt days were ſerene and warm: this was ſucceeded by ſome gluts of rain; the reſt of the month moſtly fair, and inclined to cold. The principal winds S. W. and N. W.

Auguſt.	
E.	5
N. E.	2
S.	3
S. W.	9
W.	7
N.	1
N. W.	9

The ſummer in general was healthy, though dyſenteries were pretty frequent in June, and ſome miliary fevers were obſerved among the poor; and upon the cold and winter-like weather at the end of the month coughs were frequent not only among men, but the horſes; and

chin-

chin-coughs among the children in the poor-houfe.

Colds were not unfrequent in July, nor through great part of the month of Auguft, and fome diarrhœas attended the end of Auguft, in which month fome few inflammatory fevers appeared; but thofe of the low kind were more frequent, fometimes attended with petechial, but oftener with miliary eruptions, feveral of which ran out to the thirtieth, and one to the thirty-fixth day.

Of the different fevers that occurred within this quarter, the days of termination were the fifth or fixth, the feventh, the eighth, the tenth, the fourteenth, the fifteenth, the eighteenth, the thirtieth, and thirty-fixth.

AUTUMN.

September.	
W.	6
S. W.	8
S. E.	15
N. E.	1
N. W.	2
S.	2

The fore half of September fair and frequently hot, with much dew and S. E. winds; and thus ended a feries of about a month's fair weather: the

the reſt of the month there were frequent and great rains, and the winds S. W.

Throughout October were frequent rains and ſome floods. The principal winds W. and generally high. The month ended with a ſmart froſt.

October.	
W.	13
S. W.	9
S.	1
S. E.	2
N. W.	10
N.	1
N. E.	1

November was moiſt, much rain, not many fair days; ſcarce more than three froſty. The principal wind W. A ſtorm the ſixth.

November.	
S. W.	2
W.	18
N. W.	6
S. E.	2
N. E.	1
E.	2
N.	2

It was one of the wetteſt autumns in the memory of man, and yet remarkably healthy: diarrhœas, which had attended the end of ſummer, were alſo frequent in September, and towards the end of the month became more frequent, with great pain and bilious vomitings; and indeed this diſorder was frequent in October and November.

Inflam-

Inflammatory colds, coughs, and ſore throats, were frequent in September and October, as were aſthmas, coughs, and tabid caſes through the three autumnal months. In October diſorders of the bowels became much more frequent and more violent in their ſymptoms, as the cholera morbus, bilious vomitings, and dyſenteries attended, with a conſtant painful teneſmus, not to be appeaſed without the conſtant uſe of opiates.

Some bad meazles attended the month of October. The diarhœas and dyſenteries which attended this quarter, were not often fatal, and the fevers were far from being epidemical or malignant. Among theſe, out of five which occurred in September and October, three terminated the tenth day, one the ninth, one on the eleventh, all happily. In November three boys in one houſe had a miliary fever of thirty days duration, and all recovered.

WIN-

WINTER, 1760, 1761.

The exceſſive moiſt weather continued through December, with high winds, few days being wholly exempt from either; the ſeventh and thirtieth it blew a ſtorm. The principal wind W.

December.	
W.	20
N. W.	2
S. W.	10
N.	1

January was a month of fine weather, uncommonly warm for the ſeaſon: very little rain or wind: frequent fogs, but warm and moiſt, not attended with froſts as uſual. The principal winds S. E. The barometer higher than for many years paſt.

January.	
W.	6
S. W.	9
N. E.	3
S. E.	12
N.	3
N. W.	3
E.	1
S.	1

The fore part of February was variable: from the eleventh to the end a good deal of rain and ſtormy weather. The winds moſtly S. W.

February.	
N. W.	7
W.	11
S. W.	13
N.	2
S. E.	1

SUM-

SUMMARY.

A dry ſpring, with a prevalence of E. winds.

The ſummer variable, inclined to cold.

The autumn exceſſively wet, with W. winds.

The winter very open and warm. December and January windy and ſtormy.

December was healthy, as was this whole winter-quarter, though uncommonly wet and warm, an expreſs contradiction to the vulgar tradition, that a green Chriſtmas makes a fat church-yard. Diarrhœas indeed, which had attended the laſt autumn, did frequently occur in December, but very few acute caſes; and through the whole quarter, our endemial diſeaſes, catarrhs, or defluxions in divers ſhapes, tumours of the jaws, neck, epiphoras, coughs, and aſthmas, chiefly prevailed.

Yearly bill of burials in Dublin one thouſand nine hundred and ninety-three.

OF

OF THE Epidemic CATARRHAL FEVER among Horſes.

THE late epidemic catarrh, or rather catarrhal fever among horſes, took its riſe in the winter, which was a very ſevere one, not only in theſe countries, but other parts of Europe; and even in this changeable climate, was attended with uncommon viciſſitudes in the temperature of the air and weather.

It raged in London and other parts of England in January, February, and March; and ſeized our horſes in Dublin at the end of March, moving weſtward (as other epidemics frequently do) and on the fourth of April it was become general in this city, and continued till the end of that month, when moſt of our horſes were recovering, although ſome remains of the diſeaſe appeared in June, and even July the 17th, in the coughs and broken wind attending ſome of them, in conſequence of the diſorder.

It ſeized them with a heavineſs, loſs of appetite, and a cough: a ſwelling in the throat frequently attended, and ſometimes laborious breathing; after ſome days they diſcharged a yellow mucus from the noſtrils, and frequently recovered, although ſeveral died here, as well as in England, eſpecially under too warm a regimen, v. g. particularly in the barracks, where they are kept cloſe crowded in the ſtables, ſo that they loſt thirty-eight out of two hundred and fifty; whereas I am informed that at a certain ſtand of chaiſe-horſes uſing more exerciſe, and a cooler regimen, they loſt but two out of thirty-ſix.

Alſo the diſtemper is ſaid to have been more ſevere in the North than in the South.

The mules alſo received the infection.

Early bleeding, but not late, was of uſe.

One gentleman preſerved his horſes from the contagion by dipping a bunch of rue in vinegar, rubbing their noſes

and

and ſprinkling the manger with it. Another preſerved his mare, by cauſing her to drink tar-water diluted with an equal part of common water.

In ſome parts of England they uſed malt maſhes at the decline of the diſeaſe, being found of ſervice both as a cordial, a pectoral, and keeping the belly ſoluble.

In 1727 there was an epidemic catarrh among our horſes here, which alſo travelled hither from England, and moreover preceded a like diſorder, viz. a cough and ſore throats among men; even as at Edinburgh, before the catarrhal fever in 1732, their horſes had been previouſly affected.

Again in the cold and dry ſpring 1742, was an epidemic catarrh among the horſes at Plymouth and here.

In May 1746 (the preceding part of the ſpring cold) was an epidemic cough among horſes, and chin-coughs and tumors of the parotids among men.

In December 1750 was an univerſal catarrhal

tarrhal fever among horſes, rather more ſevere than this of the preſent year 1760, which alſo travelled from England, and the like in December and January 1751; and among mankind coughs and inflammations of the face, eyes, and gums, at the ſame time.

And A.D. 1762, I am informed that to this preſent time, many of the labouring horſes who had this diſorder ſuffered ſo much in their eyes as to have become blind.

SPRING, 1761.

March.	
S. W.	11
N. W.	8
S.	1
S. E.	5
N.	3
N E.	5
E.	1

In March the weather was variable: there were ſome ſlight froſts, and frequently high winds, of which the S. W. and N. W. prevailed.

April.	
S. E.	9
W.	10
S W.	3
N.	6
N. E.	3
N. W.	2

April was moderate as to moiſture and dryneſs; rather cold for the ſeaſon, and the principal wind from ſome point of the N. or E.

May

May was rather fair than otherwise: great changes from heat to cold; so that our fires, which had been put out the seventh, were rekindled the twenty-fifth, and continued to the end of the month. The principal wind E. with some smart breezes and hard gales.

May.	
N. W.	4
S. W.	8
S.	1
E.	6
N. E.	8
N.	1

Coughs and tumours about the fauces and throat, with a slight fever, often occurred in March; and regular intermittents, tertian, and quotidian, were more frequent than for some years past: towards the end of the month and beginning of April, the cholera morbus, with obstinate obstructions and inflammations of the bowels, and bilious purgings, attended with a fever, were very frequent; and some diarrhœas were observed about the end of the month.

A few inflammatory fevers occurred, among which, one terminated by an ab-

scess

ſceſs in the throat in three weeks; a ſecond came to an imperfect criſis in fourteen days; a third, being catarrhal, laſted four days; a fourth, alſo catarrhal, laſted three days, and was carried off by a ſpontaneous ſweat, and an eruption of pimples about the mouth. Towards the end of the month ſome low fevers, with petechiæ, but more frequently with miliary eruptions, which generally ran out to the twentieth day, often attended with bad ſymptoms, but ſeldom proved mortal.

The meazles were frequent in March and April, and in this laſt month came out in round diſtinct ſpots above the ſurface of the ſkin, like the firſt appearance of the ſmall-pox.

April was more healthy than March, ſo that little appeared except a few coughs, and ſome few agues.

May exhibited chiefly coughs and tabid caſes, and ſome ſore eyes: alſo ſome intermittents appeared; but inflammatory fevers, particularly pleuriſies and peripneumonies, were moſt frequent this month.

SUMMER.

In June it was generally dry; far leſs rain than uſual, and yet it was rarely very hot, though the latter half of the month was hot. The N. and E. winds prevailed, like what is more uſual in the ſpring.

June.	
N. W.	3
N. E.	9
N.	5
E.	2
W.	9
S. W.	4
S. E.	4
S.	1

The dry weather continued through the greateſt part of July, and it was rather cool than hot, though the twenty-third and twenty-fourth days were very hot and ſultry; but no days within two degrees ſo hot as laſt year. The winds moſtly W. and ſometimes S. W. which were cold, dry, and parching, contrary to cuſtom.

July.	
W.	18
S. E.	4
N.	1
S. W.	9
N. W.	8

The dry weather prevailed alſo through the month of Auguſt; but it was frequent-

Auguſt.	
S. W.	11
N. W.	5
E.	3

W.	8	ly cloudy, and over-caſt, ſo that the heat was tempered; though about the middle of the month there were ſome hot and ſultry days. The principal winds S. W. and W.
S. E.	2	
N. E.	1	
N.	1	
S.	2	

The pleuritic fevers, mentioned in the ſpring, continued in June; and ſome few fevers with pleuritic ſymptoms were ſeen in July. Coughs and catarrhs were more frequent than uſual in June. The meazles, as mentioned laſt March, were accompanied with ſymptoms of violent inflammation in June and July.

Some ſlight cholics and obſtructions in the primæ viæ, and ſome diarrhœas, with bilious vomitings, were obſerved in June; but in July theſe diſorders were attended with inflammation, and were more frequent and more ſevere.

There were ſome inſtances of the low fever, with petechial eruptions in June; but in July theſe were more frequent, and

in

in ſome the petechiæ were interſperſed with bloody ſpecks : in others, a great anxiety and oppreſſion attended, though no eruptions appeared, but a gentle diarrhœa through the whole courſe, which gradually alleviated the ſymptoms, until the fever wore off in about ſeventeen days. The patients were very apt to relapſe, and could not bear even the mildeſt purge after.

Some ſmall-pox of a malignant kind attended the month of July.

In Auguſt vomitings, with obſtructed bowels, tending to inflammation, as in July, continued ; and about the middle of the month the cholera morbus became very frequent.

Colds, ſore throats, and rheumatiſms, were frequent near the cloſe of the month ; and at the ſame time a red exanthematous eruption in the ſkin was frequent among women, and generally attended with a nervous fever ; and the ſmall-pox were frequent and malignant, with bloody ſpecks inter-

interſperſed on the firſt eruption, and in the progreſs, bloody ſpits.

AUTUMN.

September.	
S.	3
N. W.	6
S. W.	8
S. E.	9
W.	5
E.	1
N.	1

The dry weather continued to prevail in September, though now and then interrupted by rain and ſome hard gales. The fourteenth a ſudden change to cold, which continued about a week; thence to the end frequent fogs, and it was warm like ſummer. The principal winds S. E. and S. W.

October.	
S. E.	12
S. W.	2
W.	5
N. E.	4
E.	5
N.	2
N. W.	3
S.	2

In October there fell abundance of rain, contrary to cuſtom, and the greateſt gluts of rain were from the eaſt. It was cool. There were ſome hard gales. The twenty-ſecond and twenty-eighth ſtormy: it concluded with a ſlight froſt. The principal wind S. E.

In

THE WEATHER 265.

In November the weather was variable, with a few ſlight froſts, and frequent rains. The nineteenth, twentieth, and twenty-firſt, ſtormy. The principal winds W. and S. W.

November.	
W.	9
N. W.	6
S. E.	4
E.	2
N. E.	1
S. W.	7

Diarrhœas and dyſenteries attended the month of September, and the ſmall-pox was epidemical and malignant; and the petechial fever mentioned laſt July attended September and October. Among the children in the work-houſe it generally terminated about the fourteenth day, and in all happily; and it was obſerved that towards the determination, they had a ſlight diarrhœa.

The like fever was obſerved at the ſame time in other parts of the city, eſpecially in October, and ſometimes proved fatal. In the moſt malignant, about the tenth or eleventh day, a delirium came on, with ſubſultus tendinum, and difficult reſpiration, particularly if not attended with a natural purging.

In ſome, after the diſorder had gone on without any bad ſymptom, about the twelfth day miliary eruptions appeared among the petechiæ, and were immediately attended with delirium, difficult reſpiration, and ſubſultus: ſuch frequently died the fourteenth day.

Singular was the hiſtory of one woman, in whom, in one of theſe petechial fevers, miliary eruptions ſupervened after the twentieth day, with delirium, ſubſultus, &c. and on the thirty-fifth day a profuſe ſalivation came on; and when it ceaſed, the delirium and other bad ſymptoms returned; but it continued at intervals to the forty-fifth day of the fever, after which the gradually recovered, without any other criſis.

Catarrhs and coughs became very epidemic the latter end of October, a little feveriſhneſs attended ſome of them, and hæmoptoes were frequent. The like diſorders alſo attended November, and moreover ſore throats, with inflamed tonſils, fils, and ſometimes ſmall ulcers, were very frequent ; but not malignant. Thoſe of aſthmatic and conſumptive habits ſuffered much : otherwiſe the month was generally healthy.

Towards the end of November ſome fevers appeared, with numerous petechial eruptions. About the tenth or eleventh day, a bilious purging generally came on, which continued to the fourteenth, when they moſtly recovered.

WINTER, 1761, 1762.

In December fogs were uncommonly frequent, and thoſe not attended with froſts, as uſual, but moiſt, and often ended in rain. A few ſlight froſts, and on the ſeventeenth a conſiderable fall of ſnow. The principal wind W.

December.	
W.	9
S. E.	7
S. W.	7
E.	1

January was for the moſt part dry, frequently windy: the ſixteenth, ſeventeenth, and twenty-

January.	
S. W.	11
W.	12
N. W.	3

S.	2
N.	1

twenty-eighth ſtormy: a few ſlight froſty mornings. The principal winds W. and S. W.

February.	
N. W.	10
W.	5
N.	3
S. W.	8
S.	1
E.	1
S. E.	1
N. E.	2

February was alſo for the moſt part dry: froſts, ſnow, and ſleet, pretty frequent: great variations of heat and cold this and the preceding month. The ſixteenth and ſeventeenth warm and ſultry like ſummer. Winds variable.

SUMMARY.

Spring dry and cool.

Summer extraordinarily dry.

Antumn variable, except a wet October.

Winter dry, except January; and the two laſt months very moderately froſty.

The ſevere coughs of November continued to be epidemical in December, January, and February, with aſthmas and defluxions in various ſhapes, and often attended with ſymptoms of inflammation,

v. g.

v. g. ſore throats, ſuppurating and ulcerated tonſils, ophthalmies; and in ſome, violent pains in the ear, excoriations in the mouth, and ſwelled jaws.

Fevers were not epidemical; and thoſe that occurred were not malignant, often terminating in leſs than ſeven days, and ſcarce requiring medical aſſiſtance.

Among the ſoldiers the petechial fever frequently appeared, which was favourable, and generally attended with a bilious diarrhœa, and terminated about the fourteenth day.

Pleuriſies and pleuro-peripneumonies were frequent in February.

The extraordinary drought of the ſummer was attended with a ſtronger tendency to inflammation, agreeable to Wintringham's obſervations in Yorkſhire.

The happy iſſue attending the evacuations excited by nature in the fevers attending the ſummer and autumn, may furniſh an uſeful document to ſuch as are aliens to the myſteries of phyſic, to be

very

very cautious how they intermeddle in ſuch caſes, ſince the proper conduct to be obſerved on the occaſion of ſuch evacuations will for ever remain a ſecret, except to thoſe who have devoted their time and talents to theſe matters.

The yearly bill of Dublin this year was two thouſand two hundred ninety-two, viz. much larger than in the two preceding years, which agrees to ſome former obſervatione of the unwholeſomeneſs of dry ſeaſons.

SPRING, 1762.

March.	
N. E.	4
S. E.	7
N. W.	13
E.	1
N.	3
W.	4
S. W.	4

March was a wet month: not many days free from ſnow, ſleet, or rain: more ſnow, and colder than for ſeveral years paſt. The principal winds N. W. Some briſk gales now and then. The fifteenth a ſtorm.

April.	
S. E.	9
S. W.	6

April was dry for the ſeaſon, only a few ſhowers now and

and then: cool and calm, yet a few warm days. The principal wind S. E.	W.	4
	S.	2
	N. E.	4
	E.	5
	N.	2

	May.	
May was an exceffively dry month, and the wind at fome point of the E. hotter than for fome years paft, though with a cold wind at the fame time, till near the end, when it was very warm.	N.	2
	E.	12
	S. E.	4
	W.	5
	N. E.	8
	S. W.	5
	N. W.	1

A cold, and for the moft part, dry fpring, fucceeding an open and fomewhat warm winter, the catarrhs, which had infefted the winter, prevailed greatly to the end of March; and in the months of March and April various diforders of the lungs, pleurifies, pleuro-peripneumonies, pulmonary confumptions, coughs, chincoughs, and quinzies, greatly prevailed, and often proved fatal. Alfo inflammatory feverifh colds, often attended with pleuritic fymptoms, were frequent: fome of thefe terminated by fweat about the fifth

fifth or ſeventh day: when they ran out beyond the ſeventh day, they were often attended with miliary eruptions; but ſome other feveriſh diſorders were carried off partly by diarrhœa and partly by ſweat, in eight or nine days.

Rheumatiſms and rheumatic fevers were alſo very frequent in March and April: and to the above mentioned diſorders in April, add the ſcarlet fever with ulcerated tonſils, ophthalmies, inflammations of the gums and ears, and the tooth-ach.

Several children recovered of their fever the ſixth, ſeventh, and eighth days, by a critical ſweat; in ſome others more advanced in age, the fever terminated in fourteen, ſixteen, and eighteen days.

Some mild intermittents appeared in April; but in May, intermitting fevers were very frequent, particularly the tertian; and pleuriſies and chin-coughs ſtill continued to be epidemical.

In the beginning of May a fever was common which reſembled the ſcarlet fever

in

in every circumſtance except the eruption. In the beginning, after the ſhivering, the face was much fluſhed, with a ſevere head-ach, dry burning ſkin, quick pulſe, and ſoreneſs in the throat; ſometimes attended with ſuperficial ulcerations in the tonſils, and often a crick in the neck: in ſome it diſappeared in three or four days; in many, after running out to the fourteenth day or longer, the ſkin peeled off in branny ſcales, as in the ſcarlet fever, though no eruption had appeared.

About the middle of May began in Dublin the catarrhal fever or feveriſh cold, ſcarce ſparing a family, or any age, ſex, or condition, except that it rather ſpared children. It was plainly a diſeaſe of foreign extraction, having viſited Copenhagen a month before it reached London, and London about a month before it arrived here; and it gradually extended itſelf through every province of the kingdom. In London it ſeldom proved fatal, though their weekly bills once roſe to ſeven hundred;

hundred; but in the country it was more fatal.

It generally began here with a laſſitude, a pain and heavineſs of the head, and particularly a pain acroſs the eye-brows; a ſevere cough, a ſoreneſs or rawneſs in the throat and breaſt, excited by coughing; generally a great defluxion from the noſe, and ſometimes eyes, the heat a little greater than natural, and a loſs of appetite.

Such was the attack in general; but in many the ſymptoms advanced to a feveriſh ſtate, and were very diſtreſſing, ſo that the patients were forced to betake themſelves to their beds: in theſe it began with a ſhivering pain of the head and back, ſoreneſs of the bones, a burning heat, and in ſome a ſlight delirium and oppreſſion in breathing: in ſome the pulſe was quick and low; but in general the pulſe was not quick, and even when the feveriſh ſymptoms were very high, it was often obſerved to be not more quick than in health, and generally more low and depreſſed. There

There was generally a difpofition to fweat, which ufually returned every night, with an aggravation of the feverifh fymptoms; and the promotion of the fweat, by drinking wine-whey and fpirit of hartfhorn, carried it off in a day or two, in thofe more flightly affected.

Some had a great oppreffion in breathing, who were relieved by bleeding: the blood was not often fizy, but the ferum was muddy and yellow; and when it had an inflammatory cruft, this was of a faffron hue.

Thofe who, after taking a puke, threw up much bile, generally found great relief from the fymptoms, and in fome they were totally removed. A fmart diarrhœa attended fome few with relief, but in the greater number a fweat about the third day proved critical: yet in feveral there was obferved an efflorefcence on the fkin like the meazles, or a red rafh, with violent itching, which was obferved to carry off the diforder more completely than the fweating.

Without

Without proper care and regimen the ſymptoms continued for a week or longer, and a remaıkable languor continued in moſt for ſeveral days after; and others, eſpecially valetudinarians, the weakly and aged, and thoſe of bad lungs, did not recover for a much longer time.

The languor yielded to the cortex Peruvianus.

Compare the years 1729, 1732-3, 1737 and 1743.

SUMMER.

June.	
N. W.	13
E.	3
W.	8
S. E.	5
S. W.	4
N. E.	1
N.	1

In June the weather was generally dry and fair; and warmer than the ſame month for ſeveral years paſt: frequently windy, but not much rain. The principal winds N. W. and W.

July.	
N. W.	6
W.	10
S E.	8
S. W.	15

The dry weather of the two preceding months continued in a manner ſomewhat extraordinary

nary through July; and even the S.W. winds were not attended with much rain, except on the eighth. From the ninth to the fifteenth it was hot, yet not one day ſo ſultry as in July 1760, by one and a half degree of the thermometer. The winds variable: chiefly S.W. and W.

E.	1
N.E.	1
S.	1

Auguſt was alternately fair, gloomy, and cloudy: there were ſome great gluts of rain after the long drought. It was not ſo warm as this month uſually is. The winds chiefly N.W. and W. It concluded fair and cold, with N.E. and E. winds.

Auguſt.	
W.	10
N.W.	11
E.	8
S.W.	5
S.	1
N.E.	9
S.E.	2

In June and July appeared ſeveral inſtances of the pernicious reliques of the late epidemic catarrhal fever in valetudinary and infirm perſons, ſome of whom died;

died; and their deaths were apparently haſtened by it.

In June appeared a bilious putrid fever, ſometimes attended with petechiæ; but the miliary type was more frequent. In many it appeared in the beginning with inflammatory ſymptoms, and was generally attended with a violent fixed pain in the forehead: the miliary puſtules appeared from the ſeventh to the eleventh day; and ſome of the fevers in July were attended with much the like appearances, and they proved frequently fatal in both months. Among theſe, one terminated happily by a critical ſweat the ſixth or ſeventh day, a ſecond proved fatal the fourteenth day, and in a third the patient did not ſurvive the eleventh day.

In Auguſt alſo fevers, partly petechial and partly miliary, were frequent, but moreover attended with a bilious purging, and not often fatal: they ran out to the ſeventeenth or twenty-firſt day; they fell into a lethargic dozing, and recovered gradually, without any other evacuation.

Intermittent fevers, principally tertian, continued frequent in June, and there were ſome few in July, in one of which the type was ſingular, viz. ſeven or more paroxyſms in a day; and theſe fits grew daily ſtronger, until the ſeventh day, when a large critical ſweat terminated the diſeaſe. In Auguſt intermittent fevers became frequent, and particularly epidemical among children from one to three years of age.

In July, pleuritic fevers and peripneumonies of a malignant and fatal kind prevailed much, and were ſeldom relieved by repeated large bleedings: among theſe, one young man recovered the ſeventh day, but not without a bliſter applied on the ſpot, after repeated large bleedings; another more advanced in years died the eighth day: the blood was covered with a thick ſaffron-coloured ſize, and the ſerum of a bilious colour.

Towards the end of July, diſorders of the bowels, with bilious purging and vomiting,

miting, were obſerved, which in Auguſt prevailed much, and dyſenteries were common and fatal to ſome: alſo ſome dyſenteric fevers attended.

In July the meazles were very frequent and dangerous; and the ſmall-pox of an unfavourable kind, not tending to ſuppuration, attended the months of July and Auguſt.

AUTUMN.

September.	
N. W.	4
S. E.	5
W.	10
S. W.	17
S.	4
E.	1
N. E.	1

September was a wet month, and not quite ſo warm as uſual: the principal winds S. W. and ſometimes high.

October.	
N.	6
N. E.	10
N. W.	5
S. W.	4
S. E.	8
E.	6
S.	1

October was alſo a wet month, attended with great floods, common to us and ſeveral parts of England at the ſame time. Cold for the ſeaſon, though but little froſt. The principal winds N. E. and S. E. The twentieth a ſtorm at E. Concluded froſty.

November.	
S. W.	11
N. W.	4
W.	7
N.	3
N E.	1
S. E.	3
S.	1

November was alternately fair, cloudy, and foggy: from the eleventh to the ſixteenth froſty: it ended warm like ſummer. The principal wind S. W. a few ſmart gales. The depth of rain in November was much leſs than in the two preceding months, viz. $7\frac{8}{20}$, whereas in October it was $26\frac{7}{20}$, and in September $19\frac{13}{20}$; but it is to be noted, that, although the quantity of rain was ſo far leſs in November than in the two preceding months, yet it appeared by the hygrometer that the quantity of watery vapours ſuſpended in the air, was conſiderably greater in November than in either of the two other months: the weight of the ſponge in November having been three hundred and

ninety-

ninety-one grains, which in September and October was but three hundred and forty-feven; the great moifture of the two laft months having not been diffipated by the fun, nor by the ufual ventilation by ftorms.

The diforders of the bowels mentioned in Auguft, viz. diarrhœas, dyfenteries, and a dyfenteric fever, continued through September and the beginning of October.

Some of the low kind of fevers were obferved in September, among which were fatal inftances in two girls aged about fifteen, one of whom died the nineteenth, the other the twenty-third day.

Many of the fevers in October were of the petechial, or at leaft eruptive kind, yet no remarkable fatality attended them, many recovering from very bad and alarming fymptoms: the time of their termination was various, moft frequently in fourteen days, others in fix, feven, eight,

or

or ten days: a few ran out to twenty-one days, and one to ſix weeks.

In November there was a remarkable increaſe of fevers, both as to number and malignity: they were moſtly of the low kind, often petechial, and ſome miliary, though neither of theſe eruptions were eſſential. Several of them were attended with hemorrhages, and other marks of colliquation; alſo ſeveral of them had a more remarkable exacerbation than uſual in the evening. Many, both young and old, were carried off by them; and in ſeveral of theſe the change proved ſudden and unexpected, who died ſoon, viz. the fifth, ſixth, eighth, and tenth days; whilſt others in whom the fever was longer protracted, as to fourteen, and about twenty-one days, more frequently recovered.

On the ſudden change to cold and froſt at the end of October, coughs were frequent, and three fatal quinſies are noted in the bills; which coughs continued to be frequent through November, and proved fatal to many of the aged aſthmatic.

Rheumatiſms were frequent in October and November, and ſome of them were obſtinate.

WINTER, 1762, 1763.

December.	
S.	3
S. W.	1
E	2
N. E.	5
S. E.	14

December was generally foggy, warm, and dry: little ſun, little wind, and little froſt: the three laſt days a little ſnow and ſleet, with briſk gales at S. E. which were the principal winds of the month, contrary to cuſtom.

January.	
S. E.	19
E.	5
W.	4
N. E.	2
S. W.	3
S.	4

The weather of January was much like that of December, viz. dry, foggy, few froſts, and of ſhort duration; and the S. E. winds ſtill continued to prevail.

February.	
S. E.	9
N. W.	2
W.	4
N. E.	4
N.	3

February was alternately cloudy, foggy, fair, and mild, and there were frequent rains: the eleventh a heavy ſhower of ſnow. The S. E. winds conti-

nued

nued to prevail to the thirteenth of this month; thence to the end S. W. with briſk gales at the concluſion.	E. S. W. S.	1 12 1

SUMMARY.

Spring dry.

Summer dry.

Autumn moiſt.

Winter foggy and warm, with an unuſual ſeries of E. winds.

Theſe winds having prevailed from December the thirteenth, to February the thirteenth, with want of the uſual ventilation from the W. and S. W. were attended with a ſickly winter; and the genius of the prevailing fever, as to ſymptoms and duration, ſeems to have been much the ſame through the winter as in November laſt, affecting all ages, often proving fatal, and frequently attended with bilious vomitings and ſtools, and teneſmus.

Of

Of thoſe who recovered within a moderate extent of practice,

5	recovered in	7	days.
3		17	
3		9	
2		8	
2		13	
1		14	
1		15	
1		23	

On the other hand,

3	died in	9	days.
2		10	
2		11	
1		27	

Among theſe, B. aged thirty-eight, with dark green ſtools, and ſome of the worſt ſymptoms, as anxiety, ſpaſms, delirium, and involuntary diſcharges: her pulſe, depreſſed before, roſe upon the bilious diſcharges, and ſhe was treated accordingly, the marks of coction appearing in the urine the twenty-third day; and ſhe recovered.

Rheumatiſms and rheumatic fevers were frequent in January, and ſeveral dyſenteries occurred in December and January.

Coughs were frequent and epidemic in December, nor was January and February exempt from them.

The yearly bill large, viz. two thouſand four hundred and ninety.

OBSERVATIONS.

The highly inflammatory and frequently fatal diſeaſes attending the dry ſpring and ſummer of this year, and the ſwell of the bills of mortality, may exhibit a confirmation of the pernicious effects of uncommon drought, as noted in the year 1761.

The ſicklineſs of the winter during the long reign of the eaſterly winds, and unuſual at that ſeaſon, ſhew the wholſomeneſs of the ventilations from the S. and S. W.

SPRING.

SPRING, 1763.

March.	
W.	11
N. W.	6
S. W.	10
S. E.	5
E.	5
N. E.	2
S.	1
N.	2

March was moſtly mild and dry, a few froſts in the mornings, particularly from the eleventh to the fifteenth. Some briſk gales. The principal winds W. and S. W.

April.	
W.	12
S. E.	9
N. W.	6
S. W.	5
N. E.	3
E.	4
S.	1
N.	2

April was alternately fair and cloudy, with frequent rains, and ſome ſharp weather and hail interſperſed, and it ended cold, with N. winds. Elſe the principal winds were W. and about one-third E.

May.	
N. W.	5
W.	7
S. W.	7
S.	1
S. E.	11
N. E.	6
E.	5

May was very dry and cool for the ſeaſon, eſpecially at the beginning. The principal wind S. E. and ſome other points of the E.

Our endemial diſeaſes, coughs, defluxions in various ſhapes, diſorders of the

the breaſt, and particularly tabid caſes, were frequent through the months of March, April, and May.

The fevers were leſs fatal than in winter. Out of ſixteen patients in a ſmall extent of practice, only one died, and that on the tenth day. Some efflореſcences on the ſkin ſometimes attended, and in the worſt of the caſes, bilious diſcharges by vomit and ſtool, as in winter; and ſome of the fevers in April partook of the intermittent type. The greater number held out to the fourteenth day, fewer to the eighteenth and twenty-firſt, and a few recovered in three, four, and five days.

During all the ſpring-months, agues were frequent, eſpecially in the country; and ſeveral pleuriſies attended this quarter.

SUMMER.

The dry weather of May was ſucceeded by frequent ſhowers in June, eſpecially from the ninth

June.	
W.	4
S. W.	4
S.	1
S. E.	10

E.	8	ninth day to the end: it was generally cool for the feafon. The wind moftly from fome point of the E.
N. E.	11	
N. W.	3	
N.	1	

July.		
W.	5	July was a very wet month, andmoftly cold; the thermometer lower in this month than for feveral years paft. The principal wind S. W. Several fmart breezes.
E.	1	
S. W.	17	
S. E.	10	
S.	1	
N.	1	
N. W.	6	
N. E.	2	

Auguft.		
S. W.	16	The rainy weather continued to the twentieth of Auguft; fo that from the beginning of this month to the twentieth, there was fcarce a day free from rain. From thence to the end moftly fair. The principal winds S. W. and W.
S. E.	5	
W.	10	
N. W.	5	
S.	6	
E.	1	

A remarkably cold and wet fummer, but healthy, excepting the rheumatifm both acute and chronical, which greatly prevailed through the three fummer-

months,

months, owing apparently to the cold and moiſture of the ſeaſon ; and in Steeven's hoſpital hemiphlegias were very frequent, perhaps from the ſame cauſe.

The fevers which occurred were not attended with any remarkable malignity. Several of them were of the eruptive kind; the time of the eruption was various, as was likewiſe the duration of the fever, viz. to the ſixth, ſeventh, eleventh, thirteenth, eighteenth, twentieth, and twenty-fourth days ; and ſeveral of them were attended with ſmart purging; and ſaline cryſtals in the urine were generally ſeen on the critical days, with an alleviation of the ſymptoms.

The intermittent fever, which was obſerved in the ſpring, did not wholly diſappear in ſummer.

Auguſt was not wholly exempt from diarrhœas, dyſenteries, and the cholera, but not at all epidemic, nor ſo prevalent as in hotter ſeaſons, as appears from the accounts given of former years.

A U-

AUTUMN.

September.	
S. E.	5
W.	10
N. W.	3
S. W.	7
N.	2
N. E.	6
E.	2

September was alternately cloudy, gloomy, and fair, with a little rain interfperfed; but not much, except on the firft and nineteenth, cool for the feafon. The principal winds W. and S. W. A ftorm the tenth at S. W.

October.	
S. E.	9
N. E.	5
N.	1
W.	5
N. W.	7
S. W.	9
E.	4
S.	1

The fecond and third days of October were memorable for the ftorm at N. E. and a vaft fall of rain, and great floods, common to us and Great Britain: otherwife it was a pleafant month, and moftly fair, with feveral fummer-like days, and fome little frofts; yet the hygrometer confiderably heavier than laft month, the moifture from the floods not having been exhaled. The principal winds S. E. and S. W.

No-

November was mild, dry, and fair, with alternities of cloudy and hazy weather. The eighteenth a ſmart froſt: the nineteenth a deep ſnow, the twenty-ſixth rainy, the ſecond and laſt windy. The principal wind W.

November.	
W.	12
S. W.	9
N. W.	6
E.	5
N.	3
S. E.	2
S.	2
N. E.	1

In September diſeaſes of the bowels, as the diarrhœa and teneſmus, were frequent.

The autumn was more ſickly than the ſummer, being attended with fevers that proved fatal to ſeveral, whilſt others emerged from the worſt ſymptoms: thoſe were moſtly of the miliary kind, the eruptions appearing from the tenth to the thirteenth day. They had generally been bled in the beginning, and bore that evacuation well; and bliſtering in the low depreſſed pulſe was of ſingular ſervice.

Among

Among these,

3			6	
3			5	
2	terminated in		15	days,
2			8	
1			19	

and most or all recovered.

A symptomatic erysipelatous fever was also frequent this quarter, as were coughs and colds in October and November.

WINTER, 1763, 1764.

December.	
W.	6
S. W.	11
S. E.	4
N. E.	6
N.	1
N. W.	7
E.	1

There was a great storm the first of December, as also the twenty-eighth and twenty-ninth. The rest of the month was remarkable for the great quantity of rain that fell, being more than what had fallen in the same space of time for many years. The great quantity that fell on the twelfth was not equal to that of last October the second, but both were attended with

with a N. E. wind: but the depth of rain this whole month was much greater than in that, viz. 33 $\frac{14}{20}$ inches; whereas in October the depth was but 20 $\frac{1}{20}$. There was ſome ſnow and ſleet, and a few fair days. The principal wind S. W.

The beginning of January was froſty, the reſt wet and ſtormy, with great floods, which were common to us and moſt or all parts of Europe, being an extraordinarily moiſt ſeaſon. Some few froſts. The principal winds S. W. and W.

January.	
S. W.	16
E.	1
W.	13
S. E.	1
N. E.	1
N. W.	4
N.	1

In February were frequent rains, ſome hail and ſtorms, and ſome froſts, and the month ended with a great fall of ſnow for ſeveral days, with N. E.

February.	
W.	12
S. E.	3
S. W.	12
N. W.	2
E.	2

winds:

N.	1	winds: elſe the winds were
N.E.	5	S. W. and W.

The coughs and catarrhs which attended laſt autumn, continued through the winter.

In December diarrhœas were frequent, and ſeveral of the fevers that attended, attacked the bowels.

Rheumatic fevers were frequent through the three winter-months: alſo ſome catarrhal, and a few of the miliary kind, were obſerved in December and January.

Among the ſeveral fevers that occured to the obſerver this quarter,

2	terminated in	12 or 13	days.
2		10	
2		21	
2		7	

The yearly bill was two thouſand ſix-hundred and five.

Dr. Short of Yorkſhire, a diligent obſerver of the weather and diſeaſes, remarked concerning this the ſeventy-fourth year of of his age, that it has been the wetteſt, and withal the moſt healthy, that he has known. It is true, our yearly bill is larger than that of laſt year, though leſs than any other ſince 1759 to 1765 incluſive; and, on the whole, this was not a ſickly year: for though the ſummer was unuſually wet, it was healthy, and though the fevers in autumn proved fatal to divers, yet not a few recovered from the worſt ſymptoms; nor was the winter in general a ſickly one.

SUMMARY.

Spring mild.

Summer wet and cool.

Autumn variable.

Winter wet, with great floods and ſtorms.

OBSERVATION.

The wet ſummer, particularly the month of Auguſt, was leſs productive of diarrhœas, dyſenteries, and the cholera, than

than drier and warmer ſeaſons, as appears from 1761 and 1740, compared to this and other moiſt ſeaſons, which ſeems to furniſh occaſion for refuting a vulgar and long eſtabliſhed error and prejudice reſpecting the cauſe of theſe diſeaſes, which have been ordinarily attributed to an obſtructed perſpiration and the uſe of fruit in the ſummer and autumn; whereas it is pretty clear to me, that the uſual prevalence of theſe diſeaſes at theſe ſeaſons is owing to neither of theſe cauſes: for, as to the firſt, theſe diſorders are obſerved to commence in the height of ſummer, even in July and Auguſt, before an obſtructed perſpiration takes place, and to prevail more in dry and hot ſummers, than in wet and cold ones; and conſequently in ſeaſons wherein the juices of fruits are leſs crude, more concocted, and more wholeſome, and are indeed a bountiful proviſion of nature in thoſe ſeaſons, to allay our thirſt, and temper the heat and acrimony of the bile and other juices in the ſummer ſeaſon,

and

and are undoubtedly very wholeſome, except to a few valetudinarians; ſo that the prevalence of theſe diſorders in ſummer, and at the latter end of it, appear plainly to me to be rather owing to an exaltation or increaſed acrimony of the bile and other juices in that ſeaſon.

N. B. Laſt November we had an account from Denmark of an epidemic catarrh among horſes, and that the dogs were infected by lying in the ſtables among them; and from Madrid, May the 5th, that 900 dogs died in one day; and from Genoa of a mortality among the poultry; and May 19, from Cadiz, a like account, and that the diſeaſe was fatal chiefly to hens. Thomas Weatheralt, ſurgeon, reſident at Doneraile, January 2, informed me, that there was then a plague among the dogs, which, by the ſequel, appears to have been a catarrhal fever, viz. theſymptoms were a great diſcharge of a gleety humour from the noſe and eyes, a difficulty of breathing, a violent beating of the

the heart, alſo convulſions, and great weakneſs in the back, and in the hind legs: that the old dogs recovered if they got three or four doſes of pills made of ſulphur, antimony, and tar, but that the young puppies died whether they got the medicine or not, and that it was contagious; and I am ſince informed that this diſeaſe alſo reached ſeveral of the ſame ſpecies of animals in and near Dublin.

SPRING, 1764.

March.	
N. E.	9
N. W.	4
S. E.	6
W.	2
S. W.	12
N.	1
E.	1

March was moſtly dry and fair; much March-duſt; a little ſnow ſometimes about the beginning; ſome briſk gales at S. W. which, and ſome point of the E. were the principal winds.

April.	
S. W.	7
S. E.	10
W.	5
N. E.	6
N.	5

April was moſtly dry and cool (the thermometer during the eclipſe of the ſun fell conſiderably) not ſuch frequent ſhowers

ſhowers as uſual: ſome few ſummer-like days, and ſome few ſnow and hail. The principal winds at ſome point of the E. or N. Briſk gales at the beginning and end.

N.W.	7
E.	2

May was generally dry: now and then a little rain: cool for the ſeaſon: ſome ſhowers of hail: the twenty-fifth hot. Windy about the beginning at S. W. which was the principal wind, though frequently ſome point of the N. or E.

May.	
N.W.	20
S. E.	7
N. E.	3
N. W.	6
W.	5
N.	2
E.	2

It was a very healthy ſpring, inſomuch that to one in a moderate extent of practice there occurred but one fever during the whole quarter, which finiſhed its courſe in fourteen days; but others met with a conſiderable number of fevers, attended with aphthæ, which ſeemed to extend from the mouth through the whole tract of the inteſtines, and withal were attended with miliary eruptions: they were tedious, but not mortal. Agues

Agues were frequent in March and May, but flight; and coughs, colds, tumours of the jaws, afthmas, fome hæmoptoes, and tabid cafes, were the chief diforders: to which add, that feveral children died fuddenly with a hooping and fuffocation, but no cough; and in one of them opened, no caufe of death appeared, the lungs being perfectly found.

SUMMER.

June.	
N. W.	2
N. E.	3
N.	1
E.	8
S. E.	14
W.	10
S.	1
S. W.	5

In June the weather was variable, but rather inclined to wet; for the firft fix days were fair, thence to the twenty-fecond alternately fair and cloudy. The feventh, twenty-third, twenty-fifth, and twenty-eighth, plenty of rain from the S. E. The principal wind S. E.

July.	
S. W.	13
S. E.	7

Throughout the month of July there were frequent rains: the

the ſeventeenth and thirtieth much rain: ſome few ſultry days; elſe cool for the ſeaſon. Some briſk gales. The principal winds S. W. and W. A fine hay-harveſt; but the wall-fruits failed.

N. W.	5
N.	2
N. E.	4
E.	5
W.	12
S.	1

The weather continued to be cool and moiſt in Auguſt, with frequent rains till the twentieth, thence to the end moſtly fair and warm, with S. E. winds: the twenty-eighth rain. The principal winds S. W. and W.

Auguſt.	
W.	9
N. W.	6
S. W.	10
N.	2
E.	2
N. E.	2
S. E.	11
S.	1

Through the greateſt part of ſummer fevers became much more frequent than in Spring, but far from being malignant or mortal. Many of them finiſhed their courſe in ſix, ſeven, eight, or nine days, moſt frequently in ſeven. A few others were protracted to the fourteenth, fif-

teenth,

teenth, ſeventeenth, twenty-firſt, and twenty-eighth day. The criſis was moſtly by ſweat, or by a ſlight diarrhœa, with ſharp ſtools, and a teneſmus: often by both ſtool and ſweat; and where it was by ſtool only, it was leſs perfect.

Thoſe that terminated ſoon were frequently attended with relapſes: in thoſe that laſted longer, the ſymptoms were more heavy, from which, however, the patients emerged with a little proper aſſiſtance.

Miliary fevers were frequent, and, as uſual, of long duration, but not remarkably fatal; and, indeed, from the teſtimony of an elder brother reſident in Dublin near fifty years, this city is ſeldom free from this kind of fever leſs or more.

A few irregular agues attended the months of June and July, and ſome of the continuals had regular periodical exacerbations; in the evening the ſymptoms moſtly inflammatory, and the blood very

ſizy:

ſizey: ſome of them terminated in an intermiſſion in July.

As in the ſpring ſeveral children were taken off with a ſudden ſuffocation, ſeveral other inſtances of the like kind occurred in July, one of whom (a child of a year old) died in leſs than twenty-four hours, notwithſtanding three bleedings, a vomit, and a bliſter, in that ſhort ſpace of time.

AUTUMN.

The fair weather of near three weeks of laſt month continued in ſome meaſure to the eighth of September: ſoon after rain, wind, and cold weather ſucceeded: the thirteenth, fourteenth, and fifteenth particularly, ſtormy and wet; the reſt of the month variable. The principal winds S. W. and W.

September.	
S. W.	13
W.	13
N.	5
E.	3
N. W.	6
N. E.	1

October

October.	
N. W.	13
W.	13
S. W.	10
S.	3
N.	4

October was cloudy, wet, and alternately fair, ſometimes froſty: there was a ſudden onſet as of winter, yet the twenty-firſt was ſultry. There were ſmart gales frequently. The principal winds W. and N. W.

November.	
S. W.	3
W.	8
N. W.	4
S. E.	4
N.	6
N. E.	6
E.	6

November was alternately cloudy, hazy, fair, and frequently wet, particularly on the eighth and ninth fell much rain. Some briſk gales the fore part of the month; about the middle ſome froſt and ſome ſhowers of hail: thence to the end cloudy and moiſt. The principal winds the fore part of the month W. the latter N. E. E. and N.

The fair weather, which cloſed a moiſt and cold ſummer, at the end of Auguſt and

and beginning of September, was remarkably healthy.

Several choleras attended the month of September, as alſo diarrhœas and a few dyſenteries, but far from being ſevere: on the contrary, ſeveral of them did not require medical aſſiſtance.

The fevers which attended September and October, eſpecially among the poor, were mild and favourable, though frequently running through whole families; and even ſome of the petechial manifeſted nothing malignant; though one inſtance of the miliary kind occurred to the compiler of theſe obſervations, with a ſtrong pulſe and ſizey blood, who, notwithſtanding all endeavours, died the eleventh day.

The greater number of fevers which occurred in the three autumnal months terminated in ſeven days, ſome few in four, five, or ſix days, more rarely in fourteen; and moſtly by ſweat. Relapſes were frequent, eſpecially in thoſe that terminated ſoon.

Diſ-

Diſorders of the ſtomach and bowels became leſs frequent in October. Upon the whole, September and October appear to have been comparatively healthy; but November was more ſickly, and inflammatory fevers, which ſeem to have been the prevailing kind for ſome time paſt, became more frequent, yet not remarkably mortal, and ſome of them had evident remiſſions.

WINTER, 1764, 1765.

December.	
S.W.	9
S.E.	14
W.	5
E.	5
N.	1
N.E.	2
S.	1

December was a warm month for the ſeaſon, though not wholly without a little froſt or ſnow, the laſt particularly on the nineteenth; frequent fogs of the moiſt kind, and alternately cloudy, wet, and fair, though not much rain, except on the fourth and ſixth: the fifth, ſixth, ſeventh, and eighteenth, ſtormy. The principal

cipal winds S. E. next S. W. both moiſt.

January was generally moiſt and warm, very little froſt, a good deal of rain and floods, frequent fogs, but not with froſt: the month ended fair, and ſummer-like. Smart gales the ninth, eleventh, and ſixteenth. The principal winds S.W. and S. E. as in laſt month, and both equally moiſt.

January.	
S. E.	12
E.	1
W.	3
S. W.	12
N.	1
N. W.	2

February was very cold, with abundance of ſnow, more than for many years paſt; alſo frequent froſts, and ſome hail. The principal winds at ſome point of the N. or E. The twenty-ſixth a briſk gale at S. W.

February.	
S. E.	10
N.	3
E.	3
S.	3
N. W.	5
S. W.	6
N. E.	1
W.	3

SUM-

SUMMARY.

Spring moſtly dry and cool.

Summer cool and moiſt.

Autumn variable.

Winter warm and moiſt, except February.

The winter in general was healthy. The acute inflammatory fevers, mentioned laſt quarter, attended alſo the month of December, the greater part of which ended in five days with a critical ſweat, and they were ſubject to ſlight relapſes; and in January and February the ſtate of the fevers was partly the ſame, though ſome of them ran out to fourteen, ſeventeen, and twenty days; and two of theſe laſt emerged with difficulty with a critical diarrhœa.

Tumours of the jaws and parotids were epidemical through the month of December, and continued in January; and ſome coughs and aſthmas attended both theſe months.

In

In February there was a ſudden tranſition from the mild weather to intenſe cold, with frequent ſnows and froſts, and coughs became frequent and truly epidemic, ſcarce ſparing a family in the city: alſo ſome diſeaſes of the bowels, particularly diarrhœas and dyſenteries, became frequent.

OBSERVATIONS.

The exceſſive moiſture of the winter this year, ſucceeded by a dry and healthful ſpring, may ſhew how the miſchiefs of one extreme may be corrected by its contrary ſucceeding, and indicate the expediency of a retroſpection upon theſe occaſions.

The ſtate of diſeaſes in the ſummer 1764, may be added to the other inſtances above of the comparative healthineſs of wet ſeaſons.

The bill of mortality in Dublin this year was two thouſand three hundred and ſeven, being two hundred and ninety-eight

eight leſs than in 1763. Likewiſe in London there was a decreaſe of two thouſand nine hundred and forty-one in their yearlybill; and in Amſterdam there was a decreaſe of one thouſand two hundred and ninety-one; and with us the winter of this year, as well as the laſt, was an open wet one, and ſucceeded likewiſe a wet and cold ſummer: and the hygrometer in 1764 was to that in 1763, as three thouſand nine hundred and forty-ſeven, to three thouſand ſeven hundred ſeventy-five; ſo that this year, as it was wetter than the preceding, was proportionably more healthy: and in the year 1765, wherein the mean weight of the hygrometer was three thouſand eight hundred and forty-four, and the quantity of rain conſiderably greater than in 1764, it was ſtill more healthy; and the decreaſe in the bills of mortality, ending in December 1765, was ſtill more conſiderable, being two thouſand two hundred and ſeventy-five.

To

To the inſtances of mortalities among other animals mentioned laſt year, it may be proper to add, that this ſpring we had an account of a mortality among ſwine and horſes in Italy; and in June, from Provence in France, of a mortality among their horſes and mules; and in Auguſt, from Sweden, that there was a mortality among horned cattle, the horſes, ſheep, goats, and ſwine.

Theſe accounts ſeemed to be ſomewhat alarming; and are here recorded and recommended to further obſervation, how far ſuch mortal epidemical diſeaſes among the brutes may, or may not, be a prelude to the peſtilence among men, which by the divine poet is deſcribed to walk in darkneſs, Pſalm xci. 6.

SPRING, 1765.

In March the weather was various as uſual; frequent froſts, hail, and ſnow, alſo frequent rains, and ſtormy weather:

March.	
N.	5
N. W.	8
W.	9
E.	1
N. E.	3

the

S. E.	4	the laſt week a change to a warmer ſtate. The principal wind S. W.
S. W.	14	

April.		Throughout the month of April there were frequent rains, and from the fifth to the tenth it was very windy. The principal winds W. and S. W.
S.	3	
S. W.	6	
W.	11	
S. E.	3	
N. W.	4	
N. E.	5	
N.	2	
E.	4	

May.		May was moſtly fair and dry; there were but few hot days, v. g. the ſeventh, twelfth, and thirteenth. Some ſharp, cold ones, ſome hoar froſts, and a ſmart ſhower of hail the twenty-fourth. The principal winds S. E. and N. E.
N. E.	8	
S. E.	12	
W.	4	
E.	3	
N.	3	
N. W.	6	

The epidemic coughs, noted to have been introduced with the great ſnow in February, continued to prevail in March, and thoſe of tabid diſpoſitions ſuffered much; and coughs continued to be frequent

quent through the months of April and May.

Diarrhœas and dyſenteries continued to be frequent in the month of March.

Defluxions in various ſhapes attended the months of April and May, v. g. violent pains of the head and in the ears, tumours in the fauces and parotids, and ophthalmies.

Agues were more frequent this ſpring than for ſeveral years paſt.

The fevers which attended the three ſpring-months were neither epidemical nor mortal: they were frequently of the miliary kind, and ſlower than thoſe in December laſt, the greater part being protracted to the twenty-firſt day, or nearly, and not unfrequently attacking the bowels, attended with a diarrhœa and ſometimes with apthæ.

SUMMER.

	June.	
The dry weather of May	E.	5
continued through the greateſt	N. E.	2

part

S. E.	6
N. W.	9
S. W.	6
W.	5
N.	1

part of June, though there was a little more rain in this than in the laſt month. The principal winds, though more from the W. were ſtill from ſome point of the E.

July.	
N. W.	8
S. E.	10
W.	13
S. W.	5
N.	2
S.	1

The dry weather continued through July: it was cool to the eleventh or twelfth, thence to the end moſtly warm. Some briſk gales the ſeventh, eighth, and twenty-fifth. The principal winds W. S. E. and N. W.

Auguſt.	
S. E.	4
E.	5
W.	7
S. W.	11
N.	2
N. W.	3
N. E.	4
S.	3

The unuſual drought of the three preceding months continued to the third and fourth of Auguſt, when a little rain ſucceeded, and was interſperſed through the month, but in no great plenty. From the nineteenth to the twenty-ſecond

warm,

warm, ſultry, and moiſt. The principal winds S. W. and W.

It was a healthy ſummer; and yet catarrhs, coughs, and aſthmas, our endemial diſeaſes, were frequent through the three ſummer-months.

Intermitting fevers, which began laſt ſpring, attended the months of June and July, though often of an anomalous kind; and in July ſome of the continuals aſſumed the form of intermittents.

The ſtate of the continuals ſeems to have been much alike in June and July, viz. that though there were ſome few inſtances of the ſlow kind running out to about three weeks, yet there was a far greater number of the more acute and more favourable kind, which hardly required medical aſſiſtance, being carried off in a few days by a ſpontaneous ſweat and proper regimen.

In Auguſt diarrhœas, dyſenteries, and choleras occurred, though for the moſt

part

part ſlight, and ſcarce requiring the aſſiſt-ance of the phyſician; yet there were ſome few inſtances of choleras that proved mortal, and ſeveral ſore throats attended the end of the month.

AUTUMN.

September.	
S. W.	9
W.	15
S.	2
N. E.	2
S. E.	5
N. W.	5
E.	1

In September the weather was variable, ſerene, and cloudy, and frequent rains were inter-ſperſed: there were ſome briſk gales, and the month ended with a ſtorm: it was warmer than for ſome years paſt. The principal winds W. and S. W.

October.	
S. W.	8
N. W.	7
W.	15
N. E.	1
E.	2
N.	2
S. E.	2
S.	1

In October the weather was variable, and frequent rains attended; not much wind, ex-cept the firſt and twenty-ſixth days. The principal winds W. and S. W.

November.	
W.	5
N. W.	7

In November, it was fair for the ſeaſon, very little rain: very

very mild, except ſome ſlight froſt, and one ſhower of ſnow. The twenty-fifth at night a ſtorm. The principal wind S. W.	N.	3
	S. W.	12
	N. E.	2
	S. E.	2

The ſore throats obſerved at the concluſion of laſt quarter were frequent in September, as were alſo diarrhœas and dyſenteries; and ſome choleras occurred.

Alſo in October ſeveral diarrhœas and dyſenteric diſorders attended, ſome of which laſt put on an intermitting type, and gave way to the cortex.

Several inſtances of the acute fevers frequent in this city, terminating in five or ſix days, occurred in October and November, with a very imperfect criſis by ſweat, being attended with frequent relapſes, ſometimes to a third or fourth time; and in ſeveral of theſe the bowels were remarkably affected.

Some miliary fevers appeared this autumn, which bore evacuations very well; and

and ſeveral of them attacked thoſe of ſtrong conſtitutions.

Beſides the more frequent term of three weeks or a month, I was informed of ſome of theſe which ran out to forty days, and even three months, allowing for ſome intervals between the relapſes: nor is this peculiar to us; for Hippocrates, in his Epidemics, gives ſome, though but few, inſtances of fevers whoſe criſis was protracted to the fortieth, to the ſeventieth, and of another, which, after an apyrexy of ſeven days, came to a perfect criſis on the eightieth day.

Bilious fevers were alſo frequent this autumn, though not of long duration, nor malignant, but attended with a jaundice, and a highly ſaturated urine, and ſometimes complicated with ſomething dyſenteric.

Coughs, diſorders of the lungs, and defluxions were pretty frequent in October, and coughs in particular more ſo in November, eſpecially among children; and

and in ſeveral of theſe attended with a fever, as in the meazles, but without any ſubſequent eruption upon the ſkin, except a preternatural redneſs in ſome.

A great part of November was remarkable for fine weather, and leſs calls than uſual.

WINTER, 1765, 1766.

December was moſtly dry, calm, and foggy, with a good deal of froſt. The tenth a glut of rain, and a ſtorm at night. The winds more eaſterly than uſual this month, the principal wind having been S. E.

December.	
S. E.	9
S. W.	7
W.	6
N. W.	5

The froſt mentioned laſt month continued to the middle of January, viz. about eighteen days; the reſt of the month gloomy, foggy, and moiſt. Very little wind this month,

January.	
S. E.	5
W.	12
N. E.	2
N. W.	2
S. W.	4

and

and the barometer very high. Winds W. S. E. and S. W.

February.	
S. W.	6
W.	7
N. W.	2
N.	2
N. E.	6
E.	5
S. E.	8

In February, after ſome froſt and ſnow interſperſed for ſeveral days, on the eleventh, twelfth, and thirteenth, fell a prodigious quantity of ſnow, attended with N. E. winds; the reſt of the month generally gloomy, hazy, and foggy. The principal winds from ſome point of the E. or N.

Coughs, aſthmas, ſore throats, and ſome ſporadic diſeaſes in the primæ viæ attended the month of December.

Of the few fevers which occurred in this month, one terminated by an imperfect criſis in eight days, another proved fatal in ſix weeks, after frequent horrors, and a lateritious ſediment in the urine.

In January, with the advancing ſeaſon, coughs and aſthmas became much more frequent,

frequent, and pleurifies and peripneumonies attended.

As to the few fevers which occurred, one terminated in fixteen days, with a feparation in the urine, and an abfcefs in the hip; another in feven days, with a critical fweat: nor did it appear, on enquiry, that any thing epidemic or malignant attended.

In February there was a large fwell in the bills of mortality, viz. to a hundred and eighteen, ninety, and eighty-one in a week (near double the ufual number;) coughs and afthmas ftill prevailed: alfo pleurifies and fome peripneumonies occurred, to which add the meazles.

The feafon feems to have been particularly noxious and fatal to thofe of weak lungs, to the confumptive, to the afthmatic, and aged.

Diarrhœas alfo were not unfrequent.

Of the few fevers that occurred to this obferver, one terminated in fourteen days, a fea ſecond in ſeven days, a third in ten days, and all recovered.

The yearly bill of mortality, two thouſand two hundred and ſeventy-five.

SUMMARY.

Spring variable, except a dry May.

Summer exceſſively dry.

Autumn variable.

Winter much froſt and ſnow.

OBSERVATIONS.

Here is an inſtance of a very dry ſummer, and yet a healthy one, contrary to other obſervations, having been the drieſt ſummer ſince 1740.

The ſwell in the bills of mortality on the great and unuſual quantity of ſnow that fell in February ſhould ſerve as a caution to invalids, eſpecially the aged, aſthmatic, and conſumptive, to ſecure themſelves as much as poſſible from the impreſſions of ſuch great changes in the weather,

weather, by early and rigorous confinement and good fires.

In order to give a clearer idea of the ſtate of the winds, and their ſeveral proportions to each other in the ſeveral ſeaſons, I ſhall here ſubjoin two tables, conſtructed from the accounts annexed to each month during the preceding ſeven years, which accounts were extracted from my diary.

TABLE

TABLE I.

Shewing the number of times each wind blew.

	E.	N.E.	S. E.	N.	W.	S.W.	N.W.	S.
1759.								
Spring	9	19	11	11	23	12	29	1
Summer	7	3	21	5	24	26	29	3
Autumn	9	7	19	6	31	17	15	8
Winter	10	13	18	1	19	19	17	2
1760.								
Spring	13	15	17	4	17	18	17	6
Summer	15	10	11	7	20	19	17	6
Autumn	2	3	19	3	37	19	18	3
Winter	1	3	13	6	37	32	12	1
1761.								
Spring	7	16	14	10	10	22	14	2
Summer	5	10	10	7	35	43	16	3
Autumn	8	5	25	3	19	17	15	5
Winter	2	2	7	4	26	26	13	3
1762.								
Spring	18	16	20	7	13	15	14	3
Summer	12	11	15	1	28	24	30	2
Autumn	7	12	16	9	17	32	13	6
Winter	8	11	42	3	8	16	2	8
1763.								
Spring	14	11	25	4	30	22	17	3
Summer	10	13	25	2	19	37	14	8
Autumn	11	.12	16	6	27	25	16	3
Winter	4	12	8	3	31	39	13	0
1764.								
Spring	5	18	23	8	12	39	17	0
Summer	15	9	32	5	31	28	13	3
Autumn	9	7	4	15	34	26	23	3
Winter	9	3	36	5	11	27	7	4
1765.								
Spring	8	16	19	10	24	20	18	3
Summer	10	6	20	5	25	22	20	4
Autumn	3	5	9	5	35	29	19	3
Winter	5	8	22	2	25	17	9	0
Sums total of the several winds for seven years.	236	276	516	157	668	688	457	96

TABLE II.

Exhibiting the number of winds in each of the four ſeaſons in one view.

	E.	N.E.	S. E.	N.	W.	S.W.	N.W.	S.
Spring	74	111	129	54	129	148	126	18
Summer	74	62	134	32	182	199	139	29
Autumn	39	51	108	47	200	165	119	31
Winter	39	52	146	24	157	176	73	8

From theſe tables, compared with thoſe in another work, from the year 1716, for above forty years preceding, appears the wonderful harmony between theſe regiſters made by different perſons through all the varieties of weather attending; and from this compariſon the following inferences may be drawn.

N. B. I have elſewhere given tables of the winds reſpectively reigning in every ſeaſon, to which I refer; but ſhall here beg leave to ſubjoin the following corollaries drawn from thoſe tables, in order to give a general idea of the ſtate of our winds in this country.

1. That the S. W. and W. winds are the two grand trade winds, or reigning winds,

winds, of this iſland, blowing moſt in ſummer, autumn, and winter, leaſt in ſpring; and yet even in ſpring they prevail ſufficiently to temper, in a good meaſure, the pernicious blaſts from the E. and N.

2. The eaſtern winds are almoſt equal in ſpring and ſummer, and near double to what they are in autumn and winter.

3. The N. E, wind blows moſt in ſpring, and near double to what it does in autumn and winter.

4. The N. wind blows moſt in ſpring, leaſt in winter. Thus far do the obſervations of the laſt ſeptenary agree to all thoſe made from 1716 to 1765 incluſive: but one difference appears, that in the laſt ſeptenary the north winds prevail conſiderably above the ſouth; whereas in two of the four other regiſtries the ſouth prevails above the * north.

* In Gadberry's and Say's Diaries, kept in London for a long ſeries of years, the north was far above double

5. But all regiſtries agree in this, that the S. E. and N. W. winds are nearly equal, and come next in number to the S. W. and W.

Having ſo far ſurveyed the ſtate of the ſeaſons with regard to the winds during the laſt ſeven years, I ſhall proceed next to

A review of the diſeaſes attending, from which it appears,

1. That colds or catarrhs abound moſt in the ſpring months.

2. Coughs attend the ſpring nearly as much as the winter.

3. Ophthalmies and inflammations in the fauces and neighbouring parts, more in ſpring than any other ſeaſon.

4. Conſumptions more in ſpring than any other ſeaſon.

double, ſometimes ſextuple, to the ſouth; and likewiſe the E. and N. E. winds bore a conſiderably greater proportion to the W. and S. W. than here. Hence the ſuperior warmth and moiſture of Ireland is eaſily accounted for.

5. Pleu-

5. Pleurifies and peripneumonies, moft in fpring, next in winter. Sydenham places the pleurify between fpring and fummer.

6. Sore throats and quinzies in thefe laft feven years were found moft in autumn and winter; but this does not agree to the account given in my review of the preceding thirty years above, which place fore throats chiefly in fpring; and Sydenham places the angina between fpring and fummer: but it is probable that a little more accuracy in the accounts might reconcile the difference. Sydenham's angina affects the organs of refpiration, as well as deglutition; this occurs much feldomer than the flighter fort, affecting only the deglutition, and commonly called fore throat.

7. Agues and intermittent fevers are found chiefly in the fpring.

8. The cholera morbus moft in fummer.

9. Inflam-

9. Inflammations in the bowels moſt in ſummer.

10. Dyſenteries moſt in autumn and ſummer.

11. Diarrhœas moſt in autumn.

12. Aſthmas moſt in winter.

13. Miliary fevers equally in ſpring, ſummer, and autumn.

14. The low petechial fever leaſt in ſpring, which is agreeable to former obſervations: and moreover, that this kind of fever ſometimes proves benign appears in the above records of the winter 1761, and of the autumn 1762, and 1764, compared with 1725, 1728, and 1734; as does alſo the miliary, as appears from the above accounts in autumn 1763, and in ſpring and ſummer 1764, and in ſpring and autumn 1765.

15. The rheumatiſm and rheumatic fevers appeared in the laſt ſeven years moſt in winter from this review, of which period it appears that moſt of theſe obſervations

ſervations agree perfectly to thoſe of a much longer ſeries of time above, which may ſerve as a reciprocal confirmation of the truth of both.

N. B. In the above ſketch of the acute diſeaſes for the laſt ſeven years, it was obſervable that the moſt ordinary and natural evacuation * was by ſweat, and more happy than that by a diarrhœa.

I ſhall next, from the above ſketches of the reigning fevers promiſcuouſly conſidered, give a table, of which the firſt column exhibits the number of patients, the ſecond the number of days the ſeveral fevers laſted, or the critical days wherein they terminated either in recovery or death.

* It is ſaid that at Edinburgh the ſolution of their fevers ſeldom takes place by any conſiderable evacuation: but that the caſe is otherwiſe here, and particularly with regard to ſweat, appears by numerous obſervations, which ſeems to be owing to the ſuperior warmth of our climate.

1. The

	N°. of Patients	N°. of days each fever lafted
1. The moft acute: [among thefe may be placed the epidemical catarrhal fever, the numbers of the patients not to be defined, but in thofe moft flightly affected, it might be deemed an ephemera.]	4	1, 2, 3, 4 days.
2. The next order finifhed its courfe in a period very frequent in the fevers among the poor in Dublin, viz.	26	5 or 6 days.
3. The next is one of, if not abfolutely, the moft frequent periods of all, viz.	33	7 days for the moft part, fometimes 8.
4. The next,	20	10 days for the moft part, fometimes 9 or 11.

5. The

	N°. of Patients	N° of days each fever lafted.
5. The next,	11	17 days for the moft part, fometimes 18 or 19.
6. The next, and which, according to Hippocrates, is to be deemed the laft or longeft of fevers, to be properly denominated acute, the inftances are not fo particularly recorded, though they amount undoubtedly to more than twenty-fix, and perhaps are equal to thofe that finifhed their courfe in feven days; wherefore, in a conjectural way, I reckon thefe,	30	14 days for the moft part, fometimes 15, rarely 13.

7. The

	N°. of Patients.	N°. of days eachfeverlafted.
7. The next, which, according to Hippocrates, fhould be rather ranked among the chronical, and divers of thefe were of the low and miliary kind,	15	21 for the moft part, rarely 20 or 23.
The flower kind,	7	A month, and fometimes a little more.
The floweft,	4	From 40 to ninety days.

Upon the whole, from a pretty accurate comparifon of this account, with that above, given from obfervation at the clofe of the year 1758, during a much longer feries of time, it feems evident, that thus much may fafely be affirmed in behalf of critical days, and the regard paid thereto by antiquity, that the depuration effected by fevers is moft frequently performed in feven * and fourteen days; as appears

* The fourteenth day is alfo mentioned by Sydenham in this view, which agrees to my obfervations in this

from the largeſt number of patients, viz. thirty-three and thirty, annexed to thoſe days. It is true that here is a greater number annexed to the critical termination in five or ſix days, than to that in twenty-one; but it is obſervable, that the depuration in five or ſix days ſeems to be leſs perfect, ſince ſuch patients are commonly ſubject to relapſes. It muſt alſo be acknowledged that the termination the tenth day has a * larger number of patients annexed than that on the twenty-firſt; but ſtill a much leſs number than that on the ſeventh and fourteenth, which may well merit our attention in practice.

Theſe obſervations are perfectly agreeable to the following aphoriſm of Paulus

this country, a much warmer one than Scotland, where I am informed their fevers are more frequently protracted to the ſeventeenth or even twentieth day.

* An eminent phyſician in Scotland affirms that more fevers end fatally on the eleventh day than any other.

Ægineta:

Ægineta: *Dies judicatorii optimi ſunt ſeptimus & decimus-quartus.*

I have ſaid little in the preceding ſummary concerning the ſmall-pox or meazles, having been ſeldom conſulted but in ſome deſperate circumſtances of thoſe diſeaſes: however, I ſhall here endeavour, in ſome ſort, to ſupply this defect in reference to the firſt named of thoſe two diſeaſes, by obſerving, that

The ſmall-pox raged in Dublin in January and February 1728, a ſomewhat froſty winter, after a wet ſummer; and that year there died of the ſmall-pox nearly one half of the numbers that died of the article called fever.

In 1736, when there was a very hot ſummer, the article of ſmall-pox was near double to that of fever; even a far greater proportion of the firſt to the laſt than uſual. In 1740, an uncommonly dry ſeaſon, they were very fatal in the ſummer, being ſometimes double, ſometimes triple to the article of fever, and, in the general,

con-

confiderably exceeded the article of fever. In 1743, in Auguft, September, October, November, after a hot and dry fummer, they prevailed again, though to a lefs degree; but they exceeded the article of fever in the months mentioned: and again in July, Auguft, September, October, 1745, in and after a very wet fummer, they were remarkably malignant, fometimes above double to the article of fever (See the Obfervations made on the difeafes of that year;) and, laftly, in fummer 1752, which was an extremely wet one, they fometimes exceeded the article of fever. See the Obfervations on the difeafes of that year.

And it is obfervable, that the fum total of perfons who died of the fmall-pox in Dublin during one and thirty years, was but little fhort of that of the article fever; the number of fevers during that time, according to the bills, having been fixteen thoufand two hundred and eighty-one, and of the fmall-pox thirteen thoufand feven ſeven hundred and fifty-nine, a large proportion truly, and what abundantly proves the expediency and high importance of the practice of inoculation.

From the above account of the winds, and of diſeaſes, it appears, that even in the variable ſtate of the former in this climate, ſome periods for the winds may be traced; and ſo likewiſe with regard to diſeaſes, as of coughs and conſumptions, pleuriſies and agues in ſpring, the cholera in ſummer, the dyſentery in ſummer and autumn, the diarrhœa in autumn: to which add, the returns of cutaneous and of ſcrophulous diſorders in ſpring and ſummer, and the regular gout in January or February. There ſeems to be a ſwell in the tide of the circulating fluid in the ſpring and ſummer, as likewiſe an exaltation of the acrimony of the juices.

Theſe obſervations may be of ſingular uſe to valetudinarians, and particularly to thoſe of weak or diſtempered lungs, as in habitual coughs, and to the aſthmatic and con-

consumptively disposed, to take special care not only of the winter, but more especially the spring season, whose north and eastern blasts are not less noxious to the lungs of such than they are to the tender rudiments of fruits: wherefore they ought studiously to endeavour to counteract the pernicious effects of these blasts by good fires, warm cloathing, and a proper regimen.

FINIS.

Harty (1820)
An Historic Sketch

William Harty, *An Historic Sketch of the Causes, Progress, Extent, and Mortality of the Contagious Fever Epidemic in Ireland during the Years 1817, 1818, and 1819; with numerous Tables, Official Documents, and Private Communications, illustrative of its General History and of the System of Management adopted for its Suppression* (Dublin: Hodges and M'Arthur, 1820), pp. 106–43.

During the years 1817–19 Ireland was seized by a great fever epidemic. Contemporaries usually referred to it in the singular although they were confronted by typhus, relapsing fever, dysentery, diarrhoea and many more. William Harty (1781–1854) was one of a number of physicians striving to control the lethal cocktail of infections. He had qualified at Trinity College Dublin in 1804 and at the time of writing the *Historic Sketch* was physician to the King's Hospital and the prisons of Dublin. He was a foundation member of the Mendicity Association for the Suppression of Street Begging and had practised among the poorest inhabitants of the city. Along with Francis Barker, John Cheyne, John O'Brien and others he was highly experienced in the observation of fever although his ability to treat diseases was limited by a lack of understanding of their causes and transmission.

The epidemics of 1817–19 were the most serious experienced in Ireland since 1740–1. Harty's *Historic Sketch* appeared in 1820, a year before Barker and Cheyne published their account together with communications from physicians throughout Ireland.[1] However, he had access to much of their material and his treatment is more analytical and statistical than theirs. Apart from his somewhat speculative statistics of morbidity and mortality, the most original – and certainly the most interesting – section of his work is

1. F. Barker and J. Cheyne, *An Account of the Rise, Progress, and Decline of the Fever lately Epidemical in Ireland, together with Communications from Physicians in the Provinces, and various Official Documents* (2 vols, Dublin: Hodges and M'Arthur, 1821) (see this set, Volumes III and IV).

his comparison of the epidemics of 1740–1 and 1817–19. This comparison is reproduced here.

Harty provided parallel accounts of the two epidemics (which he labelled 1741 and 1817 respectively) in numbered paragraphs. 1741 was printed on the verso page and 1817 on the recto, but he confused matters somewhat by running footnotes from the verso across to the recto and the recto footnotes to the verso (as reproduced here). For the first period he relied heavily on O'Connell, Rutty and Huxham.[1] He had his own first hand knowledge of the epidemic of 1817–19, but he drew also on information from official documents and fellow practitioners.

The first three paragraphs of Harty's parallel accounts described the weather, which in both periods was very unusual. Arctic winters and cold summers persisted throughout north-western Europe in 1740–2 and in Ireland they severely damaged the potato and grain harvests, causing widespread hunger and untold hardship. The years 1816–17 became known in Europe as years without summers as a volcanic eruption in the East Indies belched out millions of tons of ash into the atmosphere blotting out the sun.[2] Again the potatoes and grain harvests were badly affected and there was serious famine. The disease patterns were similar in both periods with many accounts describing episodes of relapsing fever.

Harty repeated O'Connell's estimate that in 1740–1 80,000 people died from famine and fever, although modern historians put the probable figure four to five times higher. He reckoned that about 800,000 persons were infected in 1817–19, with over 44,000 fatalities, although the real figures could have been as high as 1,500,000 cases and 65,000 deaths respectively.[3] He speculated that in the mid-eighteenth century a high proportion of sufferers from fever

1. Maurice O'Connell, *Morborum acutorum, et chronicorum quorundam, observationes medicinales experimentales* (Dublin: S. Powell, 1746); John Rutty, *A Chronological History of the Weather and Seasons, and of the Prevailing Diseases in Dublin: with the various Periods, Successions, and Revolutions, during the Space of Forty Years ...* (London: Robinson and Roberts, 1770) (this volume, pp. 19–412); John Huxham, *Observationes de Aere, et Morbis epidemicis, ab anno 1728 ad finem anni 1737 Plymuthi factœ. His accedit opusculum de Morbo colico Damnoniensi* (London: S. Austen, 1739); John Huxham, *Observations on the Air, and Epidemic Diseases from the Beginning of the Year 1738 to the End of the Year 1748* (translated from the Latin, London: J. Hinton, 1759–67).

2. J. D. Post, *Food Shortage, Climatic Variability, and Epidemic Disease in Preindustrial Europe. The Mortality Peak in the Early 1740s* (Ithaca and London: Cornell University Press, 1985); *The Last Great Subsistence Crisis of the Western World* (Baltimore: Johns Hopkins University Press, 1977).

3. Laurence M. Geary, *Medicine and Charity in Ireland 1718–1851* (Dublin: University College Dublin Press, 2004), pp. 73–4.

were middle-aged men, whereas in the later period women and children were most at risk.

Paragraph 14 in his two accounts concentrates on the immediate causes of the epidemics: 'the severe frost and consequent famine' in the case of 1740–1; and 'contagion' and the 'miserable condition of the lower orders' in 1817–19. A singular feature of the later period was a contemporary belief that a 'redundant population' had some part to play in the spread of fever. The suggestion caused Harty to explode into exclamation marks, but it also showed that thirty years before the Great Famine there was a belief that Ireland was overpopulated and that Malthusian mechanisms were at work to limit its growth.

When Harty turns to the ways of treating fever, it shows that the main differences between the two outbreaks of epidemics was in that bleeding and 'tonics' (such as wine) were used more freely in the earlier period, but in 1817–19 greater trust was placed in purgatives; bleeding was still employed but it was becoming to be regarded as a dangerous practice. In 1740–1 many patients recovered without medical intervention at all, 'drinking nothing but water'; in 1817–19 many escaped death without the 'aid of the lancet or wine'. Doctors during both periods, sadly, were experts at observing diseases but their ability to cure them was extremely circumscribed.

AN

HISTORIC SKETCH

OF THE

CAUSES, PROGRESS, EXTENT, AND MORTALITY

OF THE

CONTAGIOUS FEVER

EPIDEMIC IN IRELAND

DURING THE YEARS 1817, 1818, AND 1819:

WITH NUMEROUS TABLES, OFFICIAL DOCUMENTS, AND PRIVATE COMMUNICATIONS, ILLUSTRATIVE OF ITS GENERAL HISTORY AND OF THE SYSTEM OF MANAGEMENT ADOPTED FOR ITS SUPPRESSION.

BY WILLIAM HARTY, M. B.

PHYSICIAN TO THE KING'S HOSPITAL AND TO THE PRISONS OF DUBLIN.

Dublin:

PUBLISHED BY HODGES AND M'ARTHUR.
BY HURST, ROBINSON, AND CO. F. AND G. UNDERWOOD,
BURGESS AND HILL, AND JOHN CALLOW,
LONDON.

1820.

THE EPIDEMIC FEVERS

OF

1741, AND 1817,

COMPARED.

It is almost universally admitted that the Fever, which became so extensively and so generally prevalent throughout Ireland in 1817, and which did not terminate its Epidemic career till the year 1819, was similar to that which from time immemorial had been endemic in every large town in the country, and that it was merely to be distinguished from the latter by some few peculiarities, arising out of the causes, to which it was indebted for its Epidemic character. This is a position maintained not only as regarding the late Epidemic by every Physician who had observed it, but also respecting every similar Epidemic in this country of which we possess any distinct information. Dr. Rogers of Cork, who witnessed various Epidemic Fevers in the south of Ireland from 1708 to 1734, states, (p. 2 of his Essay) that "though at first view there may seem to have appeared amongst us, at different times, several successions of different Fevers, yet I may safely venture to affirm, from a series of observations carried on for the space of near four and twenty years, that no new Epidemic Fever hath shewn itself amongst us during that space :

it hath been the same contagion; sometimes intending, sometimes remitting its force: at one time more common, at another less. This same Fever hath within that space of time made its appearance *three* several times in a very signal manner; not that it was during any of the successive intervals entirely extinguished: the fire only lay buried under its embers, to blaze out with more or less violence, just as the concurring causes afforded fuel in such respective proportions."—Sentiments of similar tendency, though perhaps not as strongly expressed, might be adduced from O'Connell and Rutty. The latter, whose observations on the weather and diseases of Dublin extend from 1725 to 1766, sets it down in his "Summary Review," as a "Corollary" from his observations, that the low and putrid fever is very frequent with us, and seems to be proper to our climate; for in the compass of these observations few years, perhaps none, were wholly exempt from it." In his introduction, which abounds with many just and correct views, he refers to the passage above quoted from Rogers, and also to the authority of Boate who published in 1652, to prove that "the Fever of the low putrid kind appears to be endemical to us." Descending to later periods, we find that such of the Physicians of Ireland as had opportunities of witnessing the Fevers Epidemic in 1801 and 1810 concur in opinion that these Fevers partook of the same character with the ordinary contagious Fever of the country; and in the communications of my medical correspondents, the same position is maintained respecting the late Epidemic*. My own experience

* One Gentleman very emphatically, perhaps somewhat *a l'Irlandois* declares that "the *present* Epidemic Fever has existed in his neighbourhood since he came to that country, being a period of eighteen years."

and observation during a period of fifteen years amongst the poor of Dublin fully satisfy me as to the identity of the two diseases in that place, or at least that they did not differ more from each other, than the ordinary Fever of the country at times differed from itself in different seasons and under varied circumstances.* Dr. Barker, who possessed most extensive opportunities of observing contagious Fever in Dublin, confirms this opinion, as he states in his very valuable Report of Cork-street Hospital for 1817, that " it is not easy to determine with exactness the time when an Epidemic Fever commences in a great city so constantly infested by Fever as Dublin has been; *more especially*, when its symptoms do not materially differ from those commonly observed in the disease;" on which account he considers an increased number of patients the only certain indication of such an event. In another place he remarks that as " the causes of this Fever did not differ materially, except in degree, from those which are in continual action in this city, *so the symptoms did not afford any great deviation from the usual course;*" and again he observes that its " progress through the different seasons has not appeared

* Few can hesitate to admit that the contagion of small-pox, always one and the same, has been productive of diseases, differing far more in degree and *apparently* in kind, than do the endemial and Epidemic Fevers under consideration.—My friend, Dr. Murray of Cavan, in a valuable communication with which he kindly favoured me, (and which I presume will appear in the collection of papers on Epidemic Fever, edited by Drs. Barker and Cheyne,) states that though " the disease exhibited a great variety in its symptoms, yet on consideration I think that variety *was not greater* than we generally find in Fevers from peculiarities of constitution, complications of disease or the kind of treatment adopted in the early stage. A minute description of it would be but a *common-place* History of Typhus mitior with all the intermediate shades between that and the Typhus gravior of Cullen."

to me to differ materially from that of former years." We find also that Dr. Cheyne's testimony, given in his official report, is that "the disease has been the same (with that) which is generally observed in Dublin."

Dr. Barker's testimony, as the Medical Inspector of Munster, is decisive of the opinion of the Physicians of that Province on the point under consideration. "The disease (he says) was in general reported to be either similar to the ordinary Fever of this country, or to be merely a variety of the disease, modified by the peculiar circumstances of the people at the time of its invasion." Dr. Crampton speaks still more decidedly for the Physicians of Connaught. "The character of the disease (he observes) was the same throughout the whole Province: *it is* the Fever which is always to be met with in Ireland, varying a little in its symptoms according to the seasons."—"From the concurrent testimonies of Medical men, (in Ulster) says Dr. Clarke, it does not appear that the Epidemic differed materially from the ordinary Fever of the country; nor did it vary much in character during its prevalence, except that during the latter period the symptoms became milder, more tractable and of shorter duration."—Dr. Cheyne too, though he observes in the commencement of his report on the Province of Leinster, that "it is a *common* opinion, that the Fever, which of late prevailed so extensively, *originated* in the winter of 1816 or succeeding spring," yet adds in a subsequent part of his report, that it is "the *general* opinion, that the disease does *not* differ from the Fever which usually prevails in Ireland;" and in another place he says, "the prevalent disease was considered by *all* to be the common continued Fever the country."

110

Whatever inferences these statements may seem to warrant relative to a point now much disputed, viz. whether contagious Fever can arise from any other source than contagion, they are here introduced, not for the purpose of anticipating the discussion of that question, but merely to shew that from time immemorial the contagious Fever of Ireland, whether in its Epidemic or endemic character, has, according to every medical authority, varied merely in degree and not in kind : that it is one and the same disease at all times and in all seasons, diversified solely by its intensity and by accidental circumstances. If, then, the contagious Fever, endemic in Ireland, has at all times exhibited the same character, and if the late Epidemic Fever and those which having preceded it differ but little, and that merely in degree or in accidental symptoms, from the ordinary Fever of the country, it may reasonably be expected that Epidemics, deriving their origin from causes, nearly similar in nature and nearly equal in extent and force, should resemble each other in all their leading qualities and present features essentially the same. To ascertain whether these positions be well founded I propose to institute a comparison between the Epidemics of 1741 and 1817, so far as the authentic facts on record, relative to the former, may enable me to pursue it. Comparison is the foundation of all truth, and in this instance there is no one mode, by which we can more satisfactorily ascertain the essential causes and general laws of similar Epidemics, nor one by which we can be enabled to calculate with greater certainty on the probable character, progress and termination of such as may arise hereafter. For this purpose and with these views I shall endeavour to bring together and within the shortest compass the principal facts relative to the general history of these two memorable Epidemics; and in exhibiting the very close analogy existing between them, shall take every care to point out those circumstances in which they differed, and the probable effect as well as cause of that difference. In drawing this parallel between these distant Epidemics I shall not scruple to place on record, and in the most concise form, every important fact relative of that of 1741, as the works in which mention is made of it are few, and perhaps scarce in some parts of the British Empire.

112

Parallel between the Epidemic

1741.

1. The *summers* of 1738 and 39 wet—" In these years there was an uncommon plenty of all sorts of provisions for man and beast, which, if well managed, would have been sufficient to supply the wants of the four succeeding years: by these luxuriant crops the earth was in a manner impoverished and exhausted by vegetation." Smith's Kerry, p. 77.—" Our own plentiful product of corn in 1738 and 39, (enough to have maintained the nation for four years) was mostly exported." General Chronological History of the weather—1749.—(*a*)

2. The *winter* of 1739-40 (including the last month of the former year and first two of the latter) excessively cold, with a most intense frost of seven weeks continuance, (*b*) attended with high and intolerably piercing winds at S. E., N. and E. (the " endemial winds" of the

(*a*) The Epidemic fever of 1800-1 furnishes another instance analogous in more respects than one to those of 1741 and 1817; it was preceded by a year of uncommon abundance in 1798, and of excessive rain and inundations in 1799, by which the harvest and potatoe crops were destroyed or greatly damaged. The Epidemic which followed was not, however, so extensively prevalent, nor of such long duration, the period of scarcity having been shorter and the scarcity itself less severe. Epidemics of this description may also be partial, or confined to a particular district, as "in the year 1728 and —29, the North of Ireland was afflicted by dearth and badness of provisions," and by Epidemic Fever consequent thereon—See Rutty's Introduction, p. 55

(*b*) There are some circumstances illustrative of the intensity of this " the great frost," which deserve to be recorded:—" Ab horrendo hoc et infando sicco gelu," says O'Connell, " non tantum magna pecorum omnium strages, sed et plantarum vegetabiliumque quarumlibet miseranda lues, et calamitosa putredo suboriebantur—Ipsæ namque cæli volucres aliaque in diætam humanam accommodata animalia, præ intenso

113

Fevers of 1741 *and* 1817.

1817.

1. The crops of 1814 and 15, particularly of the first, were perhaps the most abundant that Ireland had produced for half a century, and fully sufficient for the wants of the united kingdom. The peace of 1814, and the consequent influx of foreign corn glutted the markets, and laid the foundation for the immediate distress of the agricultural interests of the Empire: their losses are calculated at 200 millions: hence failure of the home market to manufacturers and the consequent general deficiency of employment for all classes.

2. In 1816 the spring was unusually late; the summer and autumn excessively wet, cold and cloudy: the quantity of rain which fell in this year measured in the guage nearly 31 inches, a circumstance perhaps unprecedented in this country: there were 142 wet days, and these

frigidæ tempestatis rigore, denso agmine periêrunt; et quod adhuc funestorum malorum cumulum multo graviùs adauxit, radices istæ tuberosæ (battata vulgo dictæ) nutrimentum ferè constans et integrum plebeculæ et inferiorum hujus regni incolarum, a dirissimo hoc et diuturno gelu penitùs putrescebant." Rutty, in his Registry of the Weather, states that the frost froze French brandy, "coagulating it to a snow;" that rabbits and deer perished in great numbers, and also birds, with the exception of sparrows and robins. "Sea fowl escaped better than the land fowl, and the inhabitants of the sea-coast fared better than those of the inland country." Huxham's account of the same season at Plymouth is very remarkable: "Adeo sævum regnabat frigus, ut vina omnigena foras exposita, mox congelarentur; imò ac vel ipsum ad littora mare, quod utique hic accidit rarissimè. Plantæ et arbores innumeræ pereunt, vel et ipsæ duræ genistæ; vix vides viridem herbam. Quicquid aeri expositum est dicto citius conglaciat—ad ignes luculentos rigentes, etiam in lectulis algidi, adeo ob frigus horrendum torpemus, ut vix fere simus vitales."

114

Parallel between the Epidemic

1741.

season being W. and S. W.) The *spring* six weeks more backward than usual: very dry and stormy. The *summer* dry and cool with a predominance of northerly winds, and the *autumn* was without rain and unusually frosty with a continued prevalence of northerly and easterly winds. (*c*) The *winter* of 1740-41 dry and intensely cold with E. and N. winds: the *spring* like that of the preceding year dry and stormy, with the winds at E. and N.: the *summer* very hot, with some rain, and "an excellent crop of most sorts of grains." See Rutty's History, and Registry of the weather—passim. (*d*). "Verbo dicam," says O'Connell, "biennium integrum primam illam frigidissimam hyemem excipiens, rarioribus madebat imbribus, et orientalibus ac septentrionalibus flatibus citra consuetum insulæ morem frequentissimè ventilatum fuit."

3. The *spring* and part of the summer of 1742 resembled the same seasons in the preceding year: the summer, however, being long continued, serene and warm, provisions were in the subsequent winter "as

(*c*) The influence of this continued drought at Plymouth is thus described by Huxham: "Major fortè nunquam observata fuit siccitas: fontes arescunt prorsus et flumina desiccantur. Quamvis Hygroscopia omnigena siccissimam aeris temperiem denotant, tota atmosphera tamen crassa vald et fumosa quasi apparet." The state of the weather there and in Ireland during this year was nearly similar with the exception of August and September, in which months "perpetuæ fere decidunt pluviæ atque omnia nimio diffluunt humore; unde messis infelix admodum, frumentum pene corruptum, et fructus prorsus fatui."

(*d*) Huxham thus describes the same season at Plymouth: "torrida valde et aridissima tempestas omnia fere adussit: matura tamen hinc messis et opima, frumentum optimum."

115

Fevers of 1741 *and* 1817.

1817.

principally in the summer and autumnal months. The mean temperature of the spring, summer and autumn, was $3\frac{1}{2}$ degrees below that of the preceding year. The thermometer in June 1816 was at the highest 73°, at the lowest 45°, and the depth of rain which fell from February to October inclusive was, in Dublin, eight inches beyond the corresponding period of 1815. The winter of 1816 was remarkably mild. The year 1817 was almost as remarkable as 1816 for being wet and cold: the spring was harsh and remarkably dry; April singularly so, it having rained but a small portion of one day in that month, and then in very small quantity. There were 105 wet days in this year, 50 of which occurred in May, June, July, and August: in September and October there was clear dry weather, and the winter was mild and open. In September the thermometer rose to 75°, and fell suddenly to 30° to the destruction of the potatoe crop and of the late oats; in this year the rain guage measured $23\frac{1}{2}$ inches.*

3. In the first three months of 1818 there was much heavy rain and wind: then a long continuance of drying easterly winds, followed by an unusually hot summer, with a failure of the hay-crop, a great deficiency in that of oats, but in other respects a plentiful harvest: the winter fortunately so mild and open that the cattle were left in the fields till Christmas. The year 1819 remarkable for a mild spring, an uniformly hot summer,

* Among the other tables at the conclusion of this volume will be found a clear and summary view of the weather for the years 1816-17-18 and -19, with which I have been kindly favoured by my friend Dr. T. H. Orpen since this sheet went to press.

116

Parallel between the Epidemic

1741.

plentiful as they had been scarce for the two last years. The winter quarter remarkably healthy;" in 1743 there was "the greatest plenty of after-grass: the two former seasons having failed, a glut of hay now succeeded and plentiful crops of corn of all sorts, and the season extraordinarily healthful." See Rutty's Registry of the Weather, where it is stated, that there was "generally a great and universal prevalence of dry weather from the great frost to the end of summer in 1744:" nor was there much rain till the following year, when from the "spilling" of oats in 1744 by storms, and from the failure of potatoes and turf, there was great distress in the N. W. parts of the kingdom, "greater in Armagh, Tyrone and Derry, than it was even after 1739."

4. No particular epizootic disease was noticed by Rutty or O'Connell to precede or accompany this Epidemic, though they mention a great destruction of cattle, from and during the intensity of the frost. (*e*) Pectoral affections of every description and degree prevailed during the spring of 1740, as might be expected from the peculiar character of the season: these were very "fatal to the old, infirm, and asthmatic, and also to children."—In the spring of 1742 severe colds affected not only mankind but horses, and was fatal to several.

5. "In the autumn of 1740 there was a great dearth of provisions, which proceeded almost to a famine in

(*e*) Huxham, however states, that in May 1740, "Tussis vehemens inter equos cum anginâ suffocante et febre plures obruit; imò et bubulum pecus tali etiam affectu sæpe abripitur. Grex lanigera summâ macie et

suddenly checked in the beginning of September, and an unusually severe and early frost in November: the hay crop as abundant as it had been in the last year deficient; general harvest early and plentiful. The greater part of the year very healthy with the exception of September, which was productive of Dysentery.

4. In the winter and spring of 1817 there was in many places a great mortality amongst horses, but it was to be attributed rather to starvation than disease.—Among the poor, diseases of obvious debility were prevalent, such as dropsy and dyspepsia, also bowel complaints: all these complaints were without much difficulty removed under a good diet.

5. The pressure of scarcity began to be felt in the autumn of 1816, so soon as the failure of that year's harvest became certain: it encreased during the winter and was in general greatest in the summer of 1817. Famine was most severely felt in the north, and in the south west, from the failure not only of the potato but of the oat crop: the poor were reduced in many places to such distress as to be content with the most disgusting substitutes for food; to eat wild esculent plants, and even risk all hope of future subsistence by digging and consuming the seed potatoes they had lately planted. In 1816 the corn did not ripen, and when cut, could not from the continued rains be housed, but lay in the fields and malted: hence the bad and innutritious quality of

aridâ tussi maximè laborat; pereunt oves innumeræ, quarum omnium jecur tumet multum et indurescit; vesicula fellis autem, subatra bile turgida, ad enormem crescit magnitudinem."

winter: the potatoes having failed whilst other provisions bore double or treble their usual price," (in Dublin.) Rutty.—" Hinc" (*i. e.* a gelu) says O'Connell, " funesta annonæ caritas et inter pauperes populumque inferiorem immaniter sæviens dira fames ; hinc putrida plebeculæ alimenta ex pravis et corruptis istis radicibus (potatoes), aliis pravi succi vegetabilibus et morbidorum animalium cadaveribus conflata." From these statements it may be inferred that the famine or at least the scarcity continued from the spring of 1740 to the autumn of 1741, when, according to Rutty, there was an "excellent crop of most sorts of grain ;" he makes no mention of the potato crop, upon which the poor almost altogether depended. *(f)* During this famine very many perished of mere want, independently of the diseases, which ensued upon it. (*g*).

6. Early in August 1740, (in July according to Rutty) dysentery became Epidemic, "quæ sensim per totum autumnum augescens magnam incredibilemque per totum insequentem hyemen stragem edidit." " Having first begun among the poor (several of whom died from

(f) From the great drought of 1741, as well as of 1740, it may be presumed from Rutty's silence that the potato crop failed in the former, though not so much as in the latter year. I have been informed by some very old persons, that from the great and general mildness of our winters it was not the habit of the Irish people at that period to dig their potatoes and pit or house them against the winter's cold: but that they left them in the ground and dug them as they were wanted. If such were the case, we can easily account for the destruction of this valuable vegetable by the severe frost, and for the scarcity which set in so soon after. It is also said that the sad experience of that winter first led to the general digging and

119

Fevers of 1741 *and* 1817.

1817.

the bread. Though the grain escaped much better in 1817 yet the potato crop was very defective in that year from the sudden and early frost of September: hence continued scarcity during the ensuing winter, and until the harvest of 1818 brought full relief. The miseries of famine were in no small degree aggravated by a general deficiency of employment for the poor and such a consequent reduction in the price of labour, that even they who were in employment could scarcely afford their families one meal a day. Very many are known to have perished from want and under other circumstances which it would be distressing to recite.

6. Dysentery could not be considered as at any period generally Epidemic in Ireland: nor did it prevail in particular places till the summer or autumn of 1818, when it followed in the train of Fever, and added greatly to its mortality. This dysenteric form of Fever was particularly prevalent and fatal in the counties of Waterford, Kilkenny, Tipperary, and Cork: less so in

pitting of the potatoes, by which means they are protected against the severest weather.

(*g*) " On my return to this country, says the Author of the " Groans of Ireland" in 1741, I found it the most miserable scene of distress that I ever read of in history: want and misery in every face: the rich unable to relieve the poor: the road spread with dead and dying bodies: mankind of the colour of the docks and nettles which they fed on; two or three, sometimes more on a car going to the grave for want of bearers to carry them, and many buried only in the fields and ditches where they perished." One might almost suppose this author was describing Ireland in 1817.

120

Parallel between the Epidemic

1741.

want) it spread to the rich." "The dysentery raged greatly, particularly in March (1741) when it arrived in Dublin at its greatest height, though it was less mortal than in the country, to which the better care taken of the poor and of their food undoubtedly contributed." "The disease, though it abated in autumn, did not entirely cease." (*h*).

7. "In autumn of 1740 (which season, according to Rutty, includes September, October, and November) appeared an Epidemic continual Fever, which did not

(*h*) The first striking difference between the effects of the Epidemic seasons of 1741 and 1817 consists in the time at which dysentery became prevalent, compared with that at which the Fever commenced. In the former season dysentery preceded the Fever and would appear, at first, at least, to have made considerable havoc as a distinct Epidemic; in the latter season Fever had been prevalent for more than a year before dysentery appeared, and then it appeared not as a distinct disease, but as acting in combination with Fever. This difference may perhaps be accounted for upon two grounds: *First*, that the famine in 1740 was more suddenly severe than that in 1817 on account of the destruction of the potatoes by the frost of the preceding winter, and the poor were consequently compelled at shorter notice to support life on aliment of a worse character: *Secondly*, that the state of the weather in 1740, was much better calculated for engendering dysentery than that of 1817; and as dysentery, when uncombined, is a disease influenced altogether either by the aliment or by the atmosphere, we may thus readily conceive why such a difference should have existed between the Epidemic seasons of 1741 and 1817. Rutty, who was such an accurate observer of the weather and of its influence, states in his registry that the summers of 1740 and—41, being intensely hot and dry, and preceded by very cold severe winters and droughty springs, dysenteries prevailed in these, as they did in former similar summers of 1666 and —84. The same author, in speaking of the diseases of 1759, would seem to attach much less imthe city of Dublin and in parts of the county Kerry: it prevailed partially in Connaught, and scarcely at all in Ulster, where the Epidemic Fever was drawing to a close before dysentery made its appearance elsewhere.

7. "In the autumn and winter of 1816, Fever was more than usually prevalent in various and distant parts of Ireland;" it subsided, however, in the majority of those places during the winter, to "assume a more determined epidemical character in the spring of the subsequent year." See p. 4 of this work, also the tables in p. 7, and 8.

portance to the aliment than to the weather; "it is worthy of remark," he observes, "that this summer like those of 1740, 1741 had been one of the warmest and driest, so it was likewise fertile in dysenteries: but there was this difference in the two seasons that the present was a very plentiful one, abounding with wholesome provisions; whereas in the other provisions were very scarce and bad, which no doubt must have increased the malignity of the disease." In the Epidemic of 1817 dysentery did not prevail till the hot and dry summer of 1818, at a time when provisions were wholesome and plentiful. I have not been able to ascertain very distinctly from my Medical Correspondents whether the dysentery of 1818 was generally combined with the Fever, and whether in that form alone it appeared to be contagious: they seem inclined, however, to maintain the affirmative, and so far as I am enabled to form a conjecture from the description given of the disease by O'Connell, the same combination probably took place in 1741, after dysentery had for some time previously, existed as a distinct Epidemic. "Præcedunt," he observes, "aliquando rigor et horror cum calore ut in febribus fit, insequente: æger febricitat cum linguâ initio alba, progrediente morbo, sæpius siccâ, et quandoque nigrâ, magnâ virium et spirituum dissipatione,' &c. These are not the symptoms of ordinary dysentery, and among the causes of disease he mentions "Contagium ab effluviis, e corpore morbido, hujusve excrementis manantibus ortum."

1741.

wholly cease in the winter."—Exeunte Augusto," says O'Connell, "in conspectum venit febris quædam epidemica continua, quæ in quibusdam locis per integrum autumnum inter inferiorem præcipuè plebem immanitèr sæviebat et ad solstitium usque aut circiter hybernum, plures impetendo epidemicè grassabatur."

8. O'Connell states that on the approach of the severe winter of 1740, "febris hæc dysenteriæ jam recèns instauratis viribus auctæ locum cessit; donec soluto tandem gelu et accedente secunda vice sicco et aquilonio vere febris eadem iterùm repullularet, et latius sparsa omnem fere populum indiscriminatim adoriretur; dysenteriæ, aliorumque omnium Epidemicorum eodem tempore prædominio gaudens, et cum ab æstatis supervenientis adventitio calore *extra modum* diffunderetur, in eodem popularitatis gradu ad Augusti circiter exitum perduravit: a quo tempore sensim gradum reducens, hyeme insequente tantum non disparent. Vere autem anni 1742, sicut etiam æstate subsequente, febris continua prædicta regressa est; sed respectu habito ad prægressum annum, pauciores tantum invasit et adveniente hyeme penitus disparuit." (*i*) Rutty's statement

(*i*) Huxham's History of the Fever and Dysentery at Plymouth differs in some respects from that in Ireland. In July and August of 1740, after very heavy and long continued rains, he says, "Dysenteria cruenta frequens:" and again, in September, "Dysenteria plures cruciat," at a time when he states that "febres malignæ jam nec vi, nec numero adeo sæviunt:" in August, his remark is "grassatur *adhuc* febris nautica maligna, plurimosque trucidat; et haud rarò quos febris ferè reliquerat, sæva dysenteria consumit:" and in July, "jam maxime furit febris pestilentialis plurimosque demittit ad umbras; funera certè nunc sexies saltem excedunt solitum numerum." From these observations it is evident

Fevers of 1741 *and* 1817.

1817.

8. In the spring of 1817, Fever began to spread very extensively in the provinces of Ulster, Munster, and Connaught, but was not Epidemic in Leinster till the summer or autumn of that year. In Ulster it made greater, more rapid and fatal progress than elsewhere; and subsided sooner, or was liable to greater fluctuations. In the other provinces it was slower in its progress, and was universally and most extensively prevalent in the summer and autumn of 1818. It declined rapidly in Ulster after the summer of 1818, but elsewhere not till the winter of that year or the spring of 1819. The disease however still continued in many places to exceed the ordinary rate of Fever till the

that a bad Fever prevailed before Dysentery made its appearance, and also that this Fever had reached its acmè even before the Epidemic had commenced in Ireland. Huxham's Fever however was evidently of imported origin, for he states that in May, "jam grassatur febris putrida petechialis, quæ plurimos nautas orco dimittit atque inter popellum multos;" he thus accounts for its origin: "Ineunte vere (anni 1740) ad hunc portum appulsæ sunt naves duæ bellicæ; ex his ægroti plus quam ducenti ad terram protinus delati sunt, horumque pars major febre malignâ imo pestilente laboravit; hinc in vulgum quòque *sparsa* maximam edidit stragem." This same Fever continued to prevail, more or less, in Plymouth the following year "inter nautas verò præcipuè et maximè in nosocomiis," and spread from thence through Devonshire, and that this diffusion was owing chiefly to the imported contagion he thus affirms: "sedulò inquirens has (febres) plerumque esse propagines febris nauticæ contagiosæ invenio, ea nempe loca adeunte uno alterove nautâ convalescente; parum adeo tutum est recipere ex febre contagiosâ recuperatos: diu sane vestibus adhæret morbi seminium." The Fever thus imported was of a character suitable to its origin: it was of a truly formidable description, attended by the worst symptoms, with bubos, parotids, and most painful boils. See Huxhum de Aere, &c. vol. alt. p. *55*. Dr. Barker is evidently mistaken in connecting as he does (See p. *38* of his report) Huxham's Fever with the prevalence of famine, Huxham himself having distinctly referred it to contagion imported.

is to the same effect, for he says that "the Fever which had begun last autumn, returned in spring and raged through the summer (1741): and in 1742," he adds, "the summer was more healthful than the spring, and the Fever was far less frequent, and disappeared entirely in winter."

9. "This Fever," says Rutty, "was common to this city, (Dublin) to Cork, Bristol, and London, and often eluded the skill of Physicians. It raged through the provinces of Munster, Leinster, and Ulster; but was most fatal to the first, where their poor were worse provided for, from whom the disease *spread* to the richer sort." (*k*)

10. The mortality from this Epidemic must be deemed excessive when we consider that the population of

(*k*) We must not conclude from Rutty's silence with respect to Connaught, that the Fever did not prevail there also: because in fact Connaught was then so little known to the rest of Ireland, that an inhabitant of Dublin might easily be ignorant of any occurrences in that province. It is very improbable that a part of the kingdom, then neither the most civilized nor the most cultivated, should have escaped both the famine and the Fever: and that it did not, the following passage from the "General Chronological History of the Weather," published in 1749, may suffice to prove. "In July 1741, a malignant spotted Fever began among the poor, (in a part of England not specified) who had been half starved the last two years, and obliged to eat uncommon and unwholesome things. This Fever was much the same that raged in Bristol in 1740, and in Gallway" (a county of Connaught) "in Ireland, but different from what it was when first imported from Gibraltar into Plymouth, in April or May 1740" (as mentioned in the preceding note); "and probably had been a true plague, had the constitution of the air favoured it, as in some places it came little short of it, as *Gallway* and some other places felt."

close of the latter year. The disease seemed to prevail first and most severely in mountainous districts; next in marshy and boggy places, and to be least prevalent on a dry, limestone soil. "This Fever seemed, as it were, to supersede all other acute diseases."

9. It prevailed more or less in every part of Ireland, with very few exceptions indeed. In 1817 it was most fatal in Ulster, but in point of time and extent pressed most severely on Munster, on account of the greater wretchedness of its inhabitants. It began among the poor, and prevailed principally among them, though in some counties, particularly of Ulster, it was very fatal to the upper and middle classes, and in the towns the middle classes suffered much. The disease extended itself also in 1818 to England and Scotland, and was very prevalent in Glascow, Aberdeen, Edinburgh, Manchester, Liverpool, Leeds, Bristol, and London: less however in the metropolis of England than could have been expected. (*l*)

(*l*) "When the subject of the prevalence of Fever in Ireland was first brought under the notice of Parliament in 1818, and a Select Committee appointed to enquire and report thereon, another Committee was also appointed at the same time to institute the same enquiry respecting London. This latter Committee sat without intermission for three weeks, and *sought out* the best evidence on the subject, and finally presented a report of 52 closely printed folio pages, whereas the Irish Committee would examine no witnesses, and after a few sittings, presented the short report (No. 9 of Appendix). And yet from these reports it would appear that London, with its immense mass of population, five times greater than that of Dublin, had not supplied all its hospitals and dispensaries with 5000 cases of Fever, while Dublin alone had at that time furnished thrice that amount, and all Ireland perhaps nearly half a million. A Committee of the House of Commons sitting in London could not to any useful or

126

Parallel between the Epidemic

1741.

Ireland did not then exceed two millions. "It was computed," says Rutty, "that a fifth part of the inhabitants (of Munster) died. *(m)* The mortality encreased with the advancing season, and with us in Dublin arrived at its height about the end of August, (1741) for on the 28th of that month, the article of Fevers in our weekly bills amounted to 30, above double their late usual number." *(n)* O'Connell estimates the total mortality of Ireland from Famine, Fever, and Dysentery in 1740 and —41,

practical purpose enquire into the state of Fever in Ireland: for such a purpose, Commissioners should have been appointed to visit that country, *there* to make the necessary enquiries.

(m) That this calculation was not too high for Munster, (though Rutty thinks it exaggerated) is confirmed by the following statement: Smith, in his history of Kerry, p. 77, observes that, "from a return made in 1733 by the Hearth-money Collectors, there were 14,346 families in this county who paid said tax. In the year 1744, the number of houses returned were only 9372, in which space of time the inhabitants decreased nearly one-third part, which was occasioned by the dreadful calamity of the great frost in 1739 —40, and the great scarcity of 1741 —42, which were years of drought, death, and sickness *all* over Ireland, and would have been probably so in a great measure, though the before mentioned frost had not happened."

(n) Rutty here evidently means the positive and not the relative mortality: Fever was then at its greatest height, and though the positive number of deaths was greater, yet the relative mortality might have been less, as was the case in the summer of 1818. From the want of Hospitals or Dispensaries in Rutty's time, their accounts of the relative prevalence of Fever at different periods cannot be relied on as very accurate. With respect to the general mortality, however, they had better data than we have, as Dublin *then* had bills of mortality. How discreditable that there are none now, nor have there been for many years. How discreditable too that in London, where they are kept, they are not placed under better regulations.

Fevers of 1741 *and* 1817.

1817.

10. The present population of Ireland may be estimated at about six millions: of these it is computed that about 800,000 were affected by the disease, and that above 40,000 perished by the joint ravages of Famine, Dysentery, and Fever. The mortality was greatest in Ulster, and next in Munster: the *positive* mortality was greatest during the summer months; the *relative* least. See Tables, p. 17, et seq. The general mortality was greatest in 1817, least in 1818, and at a medium rate in 1819.

11. "With the more frequent occurrence than usual of irregularity in the symptoms of Fever, (such as a pulse either much slower or more frequent than is usual, &c.) Dr. Barker observes that the frequency of petechial eruptions was also remarkable; these were exemplified in persons of all ages, and that peculiar form of petechiæ, *in which the eruption resembles the measles*, occurred much oftener than heretofore." This eruption, Dr. Barker very properly remarks, is neither peculiar to this Epidemic nor to modern times. (*o*) "Bleeding from the nose also was observed occasionally, and often

(*o*) My friend Dr. Murray informs me that the Epidemic Fever in and about Cavan seemed to have few peculiarities, nor did it differ much from the Fevers of other years. Petechiæ have been a very general symptom, even in cases which had no other unfavourable appearance: they were sometimes joined with a miliary eruption, and sometimes with a bright efflorescence, and in a few these two last appeared without petechiæ; nor were they more unfavourable. A dark and motley appearance of the skin sometimes occurred, and was much more indicative of danger."

at 80,000. *(p)* No estimate was made of the probable number of persons affected by these two diseases.

11. This Epidemic, though resembling the ordinary contagious Fever in its general history, was yet characterised by some symptoms out of the ordinary course. "Efflorescentia fuit," says O'Connell, "in corporis trunco et artubus quasi *morbillosa:* in plerisque petechiæ rubræ efflorescentiam morbillosam æmulantes, in aliis purpureæ, in quibusdam verò luridæ et nigræ. Hæmorrhagia narium profusa usitatissimum in hoc morbo symptoma." This hæmorrhage was not so frequent in Dublin, where the disease was less violent and less fatal. The pulse too, though variable in different subjects and at different times of the disease, being generally quick, hard, and large, was often scarce quicker than in health, even on the 6th, 7th, and 8th days. O'Connell also mentions as a symptom of this disease, "dolores rheumatismum nonnunquam aut lumbaginem æmulantes."

12. "Another notable circumstance," says Rutty, "seems worthy of being recorded in relation to the subjects which this Fever generally attacked, both here and in England, viz. that they were generally men, and those of a middle age, and strong, and but few women; and also children were more rarely attacked."

(p) His words are remarkable: "Hinc denique luctuosa et terribilis hominum strages, quæ pestam ipsam in hâc regione olim grassantem, quoad demortuorum numerum non æquare tantum, sed etiam transcendere putatur. Cum annis 1740 et —41, octoginta *ad minimum* ægrorum

brought relief to the symptoms." I have myself observed these peculiarities in several instances, and particularly the very remarkable slowness of the pulse, "even on the 6th, 7th, and 8th days," without any urgent affection of the head, or other alarming symptom. Dr. Cheyne states that "many were affected with severe pains in the loins, and pains and tenderness all over the body, which deprived them of the power of moving," and he adds, upon the authority of some of his colleagues, that this severe pain and tenderness of the loins, which was a most distressing part of the disease in the summer of 1818, almost always yielded to leeches applied to the lower part of the spine.

12. Though men were the chief sufferers at the commencement of this Epidemic, yet it spared neither age, sex, nor condition: there were periods, however, when particular ages or one sex were more especially affected. See p. 31, et seq. "The registers of Steevens' Hospital," observes Dr. Crampton, "enable me to say that the Fever pressed most sorely on three descriptions of persons, namely, labourers, tradesmen, and servants.

millia, prædictorum malorum occasione interiisse crediderim ipse, et a pluribus perspicacissimis viris, ad fatalem hunc eventum seriò attendentibus, observatum noverim." That O'Connell is not disposed to exaggerate the mortality may be presumed from the following passage in the "Groans of Ireland," a work already quoted: "the unusual scarcity was ensued by fluxes and a malignant Fevers, which swept off multitudes of all sorts, so that whole villages were laid waste. If one for every house in the kingdom died, and *that is very probable*, the loss must be upwards 400,000 souls; if only one-half, a loss too great for this *ill*-peopled country to bear as they are mostly working people."

130

Parallel between the Epidemic

1741.

13. "It seems also not unworthy of notice that, through the three summer months (June, July, and August of 1741) there was frequent here and there a Fever altogether without the malignity attending the former, of six or seven days duration, terminating in a critical sweat, as did the other also frequently, but in this the patients were subject to a *relapse*, even to a third or fourth time, and yet recovered." (*q*) See Rutty, p. 90. Shortly after this period the disease began to abate, and declined altogether in the ensuing year.

14. The causes assigned for this Epidemic were the severe frost and the consequent famine, compelling to the use of improper aliments: "hinc," says O'Connell,

(*q*) Rutty notices a similar Fever as very prevalent in the autumn of 1739; "it was attended with an intense pain of the head; it terminated sometimes in four, for the most part in five or six days, sometimes in nine, and commonly in a critical sweat: it was far from being mortal. I was assured," he adds, "of 70 of the poorer sort at the same time in this Fever, *abandoned to the use of whey and God's good providence*, who all recovered. The crisis, however, was very imperfect, for they were subject to relapses, even sometimes to a third time, nor did their urine come to a complete separation." In illustration of this last remark, and in confirmation of the connexion between that circumstance and the tendency to relapse, I may mention that Huxham, in his history of the Fever in 1740, says, "Nil utique novi æquè certum victricis naturæ signum ac liberum valde et copiosum sputum, benigno prodeunte sudore, aut *fluente affatim fulvâ et crassâ urinâ*: perrarò autem sedimenti aliquid deposuit lotium per totum morbi decursum. Signum hoc semper est malè judicatæ febris; atque adeò hæc vel ex levissimâ causâ fuit recidiva." And again he observes, "Urina vel in convalescentibus cruda perstat ac sæpe tenuis: et licet ægrotantes pene restituti viderentur, frequentèr tamen promptissimè in recidivas incidunt."

The other classes of the community afforded but few inmates to our wards: labourers constituted the great majority; many of whom were supplied from the public works; a tolerable large share were admitted from the distilleries, the breweries, and from the watchmen."

13. "As the summer (of 1818) advanced," Dr. Barker states that, "cases of Fever continuing but for five days were more frequent than usual; and that he recollects to have made the same observation during the great Epidemic which visited the south of Ireland in the year 1801. *Relapses* from this kind of Fever have, on both occasions, been *very frequent*." (*r*) The reports from

(*r*) In an official document, (No. 8 of Appendix) addressed to the Irish Government by the (then) Physician General, the Surgeon General, and the Director General of Military Hospitals, it is stated that "very many persons have relapsed again into Fever, a short time after they had been discharged from hospital and returned to their wretched habitations, *from the want of fuel, of food, and of clothing*." an assertion evidently made in ignorance of the real character of the Epidemic, (as was manifested at the time and during the summer in a very remarkable manner by the frequency of relapses in the hospitals themselves, where no such wants could exist) and also in forgetfulness of the powers of contagion, an agent very active in re-exciting Fever among the convalescents, returned to their homes, however well the rooms may have been whitewashed. In many instances I have known the inmates of a house, which was thrice whitewashed in the space of a few weeks, as often revisit the Hospital in consequence of sleeping in their infected bedding. The influence of *contagion* is, no doubt, greatly assisted by the wants above specified, but it did not suit the object of that official document to insist much on an agency which, if admitted, must have demanded more active measures than the sub-

"complurium morborum acutorum funestorum fomes; quibus quidem latissimè spargendis et propagandis, multum favebat Epidemica *tunc regnans aeris constitutio.*" Though he very distinctly specifies contagion as a source of the Epidemic Dysentery, he only casually mentions the "miasma aereum contagiosum" as productive of Fever. Rutty speaks of the disease *spreading* from the "poorer sort" to the rich.

15. In an anonymous treatise on this Epidemic Fever, (a second edition of which was published in 1742,) it is stated that bleeding, purging, and a cool regimen were freely and advantageously employed. "On the first attack of the distemper, or as soon as possible, blood should be taken away to sixteen ounces: nor is the lowness of the pulse or the faintness any objection

scribers to that document were willing to sanction. Dr. Bracken, in an official report in August 1818, well describes the state of the poor in Waterford on leaving hospital, though at the time apparently overlooking the then natural tendency of the disease to a relapse. "When patients are dismissed, most of them have to return to filthy, unventilated habitations, covered with their own miserable rags, where they sleep in their *infected* bedding, and are either altogether without food, or with a scanty supply of probably an improper kind. *Relapses must almost of necessity occur* in cases such as these, and I have no hesitation in saying, that the wretchedness of many, very many of the poor, is beyond the power of description, and beyond comparison worse than it was last winter. Nor is this to be wondered at: it is the natural course of unremedied and deep distress. Persons who some time ago would perhaps have shuddered at sending their children into a Fever Hospital, are now found begging for their admission, and alleging not so much that they are sick as that they have no food or support for them. This is no exaggeration, but a matter of frequent occurrence."

every quarter of Ireland concur in this statement. See Reports of the Medical Inspectors. (*s*)

14. The causes assigned are, 1st, Contagion, either as "the principal or sole immediate cause of its origin and diffusion." 2d, the miserable condition of the lower orders, arising from famine, want of employment, of cleanliness, and of fuel, and aggravated by despondency of mind. The peculiar state of the atmosphere has been insisted on by many as a great concurrent cause of this Epidemic Fever; some have also denounced the "redundant population" of the island as a principal cause of the disease!!

15. The same difference of opinion, manifested in the treatment of the Epidemic of 1741, might be shewn to

(*s*) "Relapses," says Dr. Barker, "were very frequent, and at Clonmell proved very fatal;" but they were among the poor chiefly; most commonly during the summer months of 1818, and in proportion as the disease assumed a milder form:" at one hospital it appeared that "a large proportion of the patients dismissed returned in a relapse of Fever." In speaking of Waterford he observes that "the distress from this Epidemic Fever has been much encreased by the frequency of relapses, which have happened chiefly within the *last four months* (November and December 1818, and January and February 1819). Of 2700 patients admitted to the hospital in 1818, 700 at least were either cases of relapse or of a recurrence of the disease after some interval of time. Many patients relapsed several times, and such attacks were often severe: they were attributed to want of wholesome nourishing food, and of clothing and of bedding, and to the neglect of cleanliness in the persons and apartments of the poor." That *mere relapses*, however, are not to be attributed to these causes chiefly, is demonstrable from these two facts that they did not occur, at least with any frequency, until the Fever became short

134

Parallel between the Epidemic

1741.

to it, for it is manifest that they proceed not from weakness, but from fullness and obstruction. The next day, or sooner if the symptoms are urgent, the same quantity ought to be again taken away: very often it is no more than requisite, sometimes *not sufficient* to bleed a third time; nor is there the hazard in large bleedings at first, as some imagine: if it does weaken the patient at present, the dangerous symptoms it prevents makes it a sufficient compensation for such a loss of blood; and weakness, every one knows, is much easier recovered from than the disease." See observations on the Epidemic Fever of 1741, p. 10; for a perusal of which tract I am indebted to Dr. Cheyne. O'Connell, however, though he does not object to bleeding, yet very strongly condemns the above practice; "quamvis enim," he observes, "febrem hanc genii esse inflammatorii minime dubitarem, repetitâ tamen edoctus experientiâ pro certo habeo, iteratam sæpius phlebotomiam, a quibusdam *fri-*

though the assigned causes were in full force long before; and also because these relapses occurred at this period in hospital almost as frequently as out of it: thus, Dr. Bracken states with respect to Waterford, in his letter dated March 1819, (see Appendix, p. 204) that "relapses have encreased very much in the Fever Hospital;" in the preceding month they were 50, and in one week in March they amounted to 25. Dr. Crampton states that at Sligo this tendency to relapse was observable in a great majority of the patients, both among the lower orders and the higher classes since the *short* Fever became the prevailing form of the disease: he adds that the Physicians of Sligo were unable to assign any particular cause for this change in the period and form of the Epidemic. Dr. Cheyne too states that the tendency to relapse was much more frequent in the decline of the Epidemic than at the commencement or during its height. He adds that, "*it is thought,*" relapses have been less frequent since the convalescents were supplied with nourishment.

135

Fevers of 1741 *and* 1817.

1817.

exist (almost *totidem verbis*) in that of 1817, especially as regards the more active measures of the antiphlogistic plan. In both Epidemics a cool regimen was observed, and with marked benefit; and it must appear not a little singular that in the remedial plan laid down for the Fever of 1741 we find so little mention made of wine, bark, and of other tonics and stimulants from which our practice has been so lately emancipated. Dr. Barker, than whom few are possessed of more extensive experience in Fever, or better qualified to profit by it, employed in cases of delirium or phrenitic action cold applications, leeches, section of the temporal artery, or venesection, as the urgency of symptoms might require. " Wine," he observes, " is given more sparingly in Cork-street hospital than it formerly was, and, so far as I can judge, the change is beneficial." " In *every* case the alvine evacuations were attended to, and purgatives directed to procure a sufficiently lax state of the bowels." Dr. Cheyne, who admits himself the advocate for " discriminative blood-letting" in Fever, seldom exceeded 12 oz. at one bleeding, 10 oz. being the average quantity: from his tables it appears that of 701 patients, 371 were blooded, 77 of them twice, 16 three times, 9 four times, 1 five times, and 1 six times, the deaths being 43. (*t*) It would appear, however, that in

(*t*) Dr. Cheyne states that " of about 300 patients admitted in April, May, June, July, and August, (1817) 149 were let blood, some of these three or four times. Of these, immediate relief after blood-letting was experienced by 94, but I am convinced that a much greater number were in an improved state on the day after they were bled." " Bleeding did not appear to me injurious in any one instance in which it was performed

136

Parallel between the Epidemic

1741.

gidi nimium regiminis patronis eo nomine institutam, ut massæ sanguineæ scilicet inflammatio, *hujusce febris*, ut aiunt, *causa unica* tollatur, haud adeo feliciter cessisse;" &c. O'Connell himself bled in the commencement of the disease to ten ounces, and if delirium or phrenitis set in, opened the jugular vein, yet he adds that neither these means "nec alia quoque methodus antiphlogistica, horrendam huic febri supervenientem phrenitidem aut vigilias pertinaces reprimere valeant." It is very evident, however, on an examination of his practice, that he neglected the alvine evacuation quite too much, relying as he did on an emetic and an occasional enema, apparently under greater fears of purging than of bleeding: hence we cannot feel surprise at the frequent occurrence of the "horrenda phrenitis." In p. 338, et seq. he gives some satisfactory reasons for considering the disease of an inflammatory type, or rather, to use his own words, "peculiaris cujusdam inflammationis fuisse participem." Among other circumstances, he mentions two facts, well worthy of attention, though little acted on till later days: "experientiâ quotidianâ constabat ægros (he says) præ delirio phrenitico furentes, qui a lecto invitis nutricibus nudi surrexerunt, et se liberiori auræ exposuerunt, (nullo omninò indè damno recepto,) a phrenitide tamen istâ horrendâ, hoc fortuito casu haud parum sublevatos fuisse." "Pauperes etiam eâdem febre decumbentes phrenetici facti,

in my wards. Blood-letting was several times employed as a part of the euthanasia, when perhaps it shortened the patient's life by a few hours, but of this I am by no means certain."

Fevers of 1741 *and* 1817.

1817.

other parts of Ireland venesection was found either unnecessary or injurious. Thus, Dr. Mawe says that "at Tralee he has in hospital practice discarded almost every medicine, except purgatives and emetics, and that the event justifies him: in 1300 cases he does not recollect to have employed the lancet three times." See Appendix, p. 229. My friend Dr. Murray, with whose very judicious treatment of disease I am well acquainted, states that at Cavan "bleeding did not form a part of our general practice, and I verily believe that none of our patients died for want of it: three of those who died of Fever (uncomplicated) had been bled before admission." (*u*) Dr. Bracken too, the soundness of whose medical judgment those who know him will never call in question, states in his report for Waterford that, "I have it not in my power to say whether bleeding be useful or injurious in this Epidemic, as I did not resort to

(*u*) Let it not be inferred from this remark, that Dr. Murray, though fearful of the abuse of this valuable remedy, is therefore hostile to bleeding in every case of Fever. In the valuable communication, with which I have been favoured by him, will be found many remarks on this subject, indicative of that sound and discriminating judgment for which he has ever been distinguished. "Bleeding," he observes, "is a remedy of which we cannot say generally (as we can of many others) that if it does no good, it will do no harm; and at a time when the medical rage seems to be so much for *bold* practice, they who have acquired a kind of authority in the profession ought to be cautious how they recommend in too strong terms a practice *which is very liable to abuse.* Other remedies may by their sensible operation give timely notice of their danger: the ill effects of this, when used improperly or carried too far, are often irreparable." "The advocates of this practice have indeed furnished strong, or rather plausible evidence in its support, and I cannot discredit some of their practical reports, but they have

138

Parallel between the Epidemic

1741.

aquæ communis liberaliori potu, absque vel minimo regiminis aut remediorum apparatu, a phrenitide et febre liberati, frequentèr evaserunt." "Many of the poor, says Rutty, "abandoned through necessity to a low acescent diet, and some of them drinking nothing but water, recovered." From an observation in Short's Chronological History it would appear as if bleeding and blisters had been very destructive in this Epidemic at Galway: "they and bleeding," he says, "had made doubly fine work of it."

evidently over-rated its value, and given *altogether to it* the credit due to their purgatives, which were constantly and actively administered at the same time." "Of topical bleeding I think very differently; this is in many cases a valuable and necessary remedy. To Dr. Mills the medical profession is greatly indebted for fixing attention on the topical characters (or what I would call the *topical effects*) of Fever. One great point in the treatment should be to preserve a due ballance in the circulating system; as the chief source of danger arises from the force of the disease falling on particular organs; from the irregularity, rather than from the general violence of Fever. Hence we often find the head or chest severely affected when the extremities are cold, and when there is neither general plethora nor inflammatory diathesis. For many reasons the brain is most likely to suffer in this way; the unyielding nature of its bony case; the direct force of the heart's action; the recumbent posture; all conspire to make it suffer. On this account, I think too much stress cannot be laid on the necessity of bleeding from the head, when other means are not sufficient to relieve it. But I cannot help fearing the practical bad consequences of a doctrine, which makes the essence of Fever consist in an inflammation."

Fevers of 1741 *and* 1817.

1817.

it in any case, and I must say that I do not regret it was not resorted to in any of the fatal cases under my care." Dr. Bracken remarks at the same time, that "wine was very generally made use of, and with the best effects." *(v)* In Cork too, I should conjecture that blood-letting was not much resorted to, as from the quantity of wine used in the Fever Hospitals of that city, and from the small mortality in them, that medicine would appear, at least, not to have been injurious. *(w)* We know also full well that in this Epidemic, if many have escaped death by the aid of the lancet and of wine, thousands recovered without the help of either.

(v) It is generally understood that the inhabitants of the south of Ireland, and particularly of Waterford, do not bear blood-letting, even in inflammatory diseases, at all so well as their more northern neighbours. May not such local peculiarities account for much difference of opinion among medical men on particular points of practice?

(w) The great consumption of wine in the Cork hospital is proved by the application made to the Commissioners of the Revenue to import it duty free; and though the inference may appear reasonable that bleeding was neither much employed nor much required, where wine was used to such extent as to render that application expedient, yet I find by a communication received from Dr. Barry since this sheet was sent to press, that "venesection was very extensively practised in the Cork Fever Hospital, both before and during the Epidemic, being eminently useful both in mitigating and shortening the disease. The quantity of blood drawn in the numerous cases of synochus, with which our hospital was crowded, varied from six to ten or twelve ounces; in my practice I generally preferred repeated small bleedings in the mode recommended by Dr. Mills. My friend and brother Physician, Dr. Beamish, generally preferred the larger quantity to commence with. It would require too long a detail to enter into my reasons for the difference. I must, however, in justice to Dr. Beamish say, that his practice of venesection was judicious and useful, and I think I observed that one bleeding was often sufficient in his mode; where it sometimes required to be repeated two or three times in the manner prescribed by me; the ultimate results were, however, the same. Local

140

From the foregoing comparison of these two very remarkable Epidemic seasons it appears that they agreed in the following particulars:—viz.

1*st.* In being immediately preceded by years of great abundance, and also in being followed by plentiful years, "extraordinarily healthful." 2*d.* In being exempt from any Epizootic disease. 3*d.* In being attended by great

bleedings were practised by us both with decided benefit. While on this subject, I should remark farther that where I have been called in at an early period, in private practice particularly, I have checked the progress of the disease in its most threatening form by *very extensive venesection.*

Dr. Beamish and myself have been compelled to use wine in the cases of low Typhus, which formed a great proportion of the inmates of the hospital. Our plan of administering wine was to give it in cases of great debility, till the strength was restored, and then gradually to diminish the quantity. From the low state in which many of the patients were brought into the hospital, we were under the necessity of directing a considerable quantity of wine, as it was in fact the only stimulant which seemed to have durable effects; but compared with other similar institutions, the wine used in the Cork House of Recovery was, I have reason to believe, very moderate in quantity."—I find also I was mistaken in my supposition that the services of the Medical Inspectors at Cork were unbought. The Managing Committees of their Fever Hospitals, however, when they determined not to accept the gratuitous services of the Physicians, would not degrade the profession, as in Dublin, by fixing a rate of renumeration, equal to brick-layers wages: the Inspectors received fifteen guineas per month, and appear to have performed their duty in the most active and exemplary manner, though with little permanent benefit, from the want of an efficient controlling power to carry their suggestions into effect. I further find that, besides the instructions given to the Committee of Physicians, as stated in p. 92, they were also directed "to resort to such other measures as may appear necessary to ascertain the extent and nature of the Epidemic Fever:" this addition to their instructions renders it still more extraordinary that they should neglect every other mode of deriving information, but that which a short inspection of the hospitals afforded them. It has also been stated to me that Dr. Rogers' name, as subscribed to the report, p. 94, instead of Jeremiah, should be Joseph P. Rogers.

scarcity, amounting almost to famine, which continued for about a year and a-half in the Epidemic of 1741, and for a term somewhat longer in that of 1817. *4th.* In being attended by Fever and Dysentery as the reigning, and almost exclusive Epidemics of the island: these diseases appearing both in a distinct and combined form, and superseding other acute affections.

The Epidemic Fevers also of these seasons agreed in the following particulars: viz.

1st. In their commencement, duration, and progress; each having commenced partially in the autumn of the first year of scarcity; having subsided during the following winter, and in the subsequent year spread over the whole island: that of 1741 continuing about two years, and that of 1817 about two years and a half, upon an average of the whole island.

2d. In their characteristic symptoms, causes, and general treatment: in all which respects their coincidence was very remarkable, as also, *3d.* In changing, when at their greatest height, to a short Fever of 5 or 7 days duration, with a remarkable tendency to relapse; such change having in both Epidemics immediately preceded the gradual subsidence of each.

From the same comparison it appears that these Epidemic seasons differed in the following circumstances:—viz.

1st. And most *remarkably* in the weather peculiar to each: that of 1741 being characterised by two very severe winters, and two very dry summers, one of which was very hot: that of 1817 was equally characterised by mild winters, and very wet and cool summers.*

2d. The Dysentery of 1741 preceded the appearance of the Fever, the summer of 1740 being remarkably dry and partially hot, whereas during the late Epidemic season Fever had prevailed for more than one year

* From this very remarkable difference between two Epidemic seasons productive of similar diseases, this inference is obvious, that the state of the weather exerted no *direct* influence in producing the Epidemic Fever of either year, that influence being, as Rutty terms it, merely "*consequential*" in its operation on the harvest. The very dry, as well as the very wet summer, was equally destructive to the produce of the earth, and both kinds of weather, however strongly opposed, were equally instrumental in exciting Epidemic Fever through the medium of famine and its effects. Dr. Rutty, upon the *honesty* of whose observations every reliance may, I believe, be placed, in the introduction to his history of the weather gives a table of the mortality in Dublin during dry and wet years, from whence it would appear that the former were far more unhealthy than the latter. From this fact certain *unqualified* positions have latterly been advanced respecting the influence of wet seasons, which Rutty has by no means sanctioned. Dr. Percival in his paper on the Epidemic Fevers of Dublin has stated, on the authority of Dr. Quin, (who took the fact from Rutty) that "protracted dry weather is peculiarly productive of Fever in Dublin and that rainy weather, which is the prevalent character of the climate, agrees best with the general health of its inhabitants." Dr. Cheyne, relying on this dictum, observes that "the Fever of 1817 appeared to be unconnected with any peculiar condition of the atmosphere, the summer having been wet and cold, and *wet and cold summers*, as I have observed on a former occasion, being counted healthy ones in Dublin." Now Rutty is so far from sanctioning such an inference, that he distinctly qualifies his own position by this observation: "we are not, he says, to understand by this but that excessive and long continued rains and moisture," (such as we had in 1816 and —17) "are also unwholesome and productive of diseases, as well as excessive drought; for it has appeared upon a review of a long series of years, that of excessive rainy years, three out of four were Epidemic and mortal, especially when attended with S. or S. W. winds; and *that they have this effect*, not always *primarily*, but *consequentially*, as they *corrupt and spoil the fruits of the earth*." That this was the case in 1816 and — 7, we must all well remember: I have already mentioned that the Epidemic Fever of 1800 —1801 was imme-

before Dysentery shewed itself in the hot and dry summer of 1818. See note to p. 120.

3d. Though both Epidemics were extensively prevalent and very destructive, yet that of 1741 was much more fatal, as it would appear that in a populatiou of two millions one of every 25 perished, while in the late Epidemic perhaps not more than 1 in 130.

4th. These Fevers also differed in the subjects attacked: men of a middle age being the chief sufferers in the first, while women and children suffered in large proportion during the latter Epidemic.

In the subsequent and concluding chapter on the causes, medical and statistical, which expose Ireland to frequent and severe visitations of Epidemic Fever I shall make such use of these, and of the other facts already detailed, as they may seem reasonably to warrant.

diately preceded by a summer and autumn of excessive wetness, and followed by a season of great scarcity. Dr. Rogers too in his essay on the Epidemic diseases of Cork states that, "during the particular series of years that Epidemic disorders have reigned most amongst us, the several seasons were remarkable for moisture and warmth:" and in another place he observes that "the particular years, most signal for the production of Small-pox, Dysenteries and Fevers, were attended with cold and moist summers, and warm and moist winters." Under all these circumstances, therefore, Rutty will appear fully warranted in the assertion that "whenever we observe the usual harmony and proportion of the winds and attendant weather to vary *much*, we may expect an unhealthy season, as was notoriously the case in the excessive moist seasons, preceding the great frost in 1740, and the no less unusually dry season, and long continuance of N. E. Winds, succeeding the great frost for some years;" "which," as he piously adds, "although necessary afflicting dispensations and chastisements of a stupid and sinful world, we have cause to acknowledge have been dealt out to us with a very gentle hand." See his Registry of the Weather, p. 418.

Bibliography

[Jonathan Swift], *A Short View of the State of Ireland* (1727–8)

Primary:

[Jonathan Swift], *A Short View of the State of Ireland* (Dublin: S. Harding, 1727–8).

[Jonathan Swift], *An Answer to a Paper, called A Memorial of the Poor Inhabitants, Tradesmen and Labourers of the Kingdom of Ireland. By the Author of the Short View of the State of Ireland* (Dublin: S. Harding, 1728)

[Anon], *The Memorial of the Poor Inhabitants, Tradesmen, and Labourers of the Kingdom of Ireland* (Dublin: S. Harding, 1728).

Secondary:

David Arnold, *Famine; Social Crisis and Historical Change* (Oxford: B. Blackwell, 1988).

J.C. Beckett, 'Literature in English, 1691–1800' in T.W. Moody and W.E. Vaughan (eds), *A New History of Ireland*, vol. IV, *Eighteenth-Century Ireland, 1691–1800* (Oxford: Clarendon Press, 1986), pp. 424–70.

L.A. Clarkson and E. Margaret Crawford, *Feast and Famine: A History of Food and Nutrition in Ireland 1500–1920* (Oxford: Oxford University Press, 2001).

L.M. Cullen, 'Economic Development, 1691–1750' in T.W. Moody and W.E. Vaughan (eds), *A New History of Ireland*, vol. IV, *Eighteenth-Century Ireland, 1691–1800* (Oxford: Clarendon Press, 1986), pp. 123–58.

Herbert Davies (ed.), *Jonathan Swift, Irish Tracts 1728–1733* (Oxford: Oxford University Press, 1955).

E.M. Johnston-Liik, 'Whitshed, William (1679–1727)', *Oxford Dictionary of National Biography (ODNB)* (Oxford: Oxford University Press, 2004).

Clive Probyn, 'Swift, Jonathan (1667–1745)', *Oxford Dictionary of National Biography (ODNB)* (Oxford: Oxford University Press, 2004).

James D. Woolley (ed.), *Jonathan Swift and Thomas Sheridan: The Intelligencer* (Oxford: Oxford University Press, 1992).

John Rutty, *A Chronological History of the Weather and Seasons, and of the Prevailing Diseases in Dublin* (1770)

Primary:
John Rutty, *A Chronological History of the Weather and Seasons, and of the Prevailing Diseases in Dublin. With their Various Periods, Successions, and Revolutions, during the Space of Forty Years. With a Comparative View of the Difference of the Irish Climate and Diseases, and those of England and other Countries* (London: Robinson and Roberts, 1770).

Secondary:
C.S. Breathnach, 'Doctor John Rutty [1698–1777]: Medicine and Meteorology', *Journal of the Irish Colleges of Physicians and Surgeons*, 29:2 (2000), pp. 106–8.
David Dickson, *Arctic Ireland. The Extraordinary Story of the Great Frost and Forgotten Famine of 1740–41* (Belfast: White Row Press, 1997).
Jan Golinski, 'Putting the Weather in Order: Narrative and Discipline in Eighteenth-Century Weather Diaries'. Paper given at the William Andrews Clark Memorial Library, UCLA, Los Angeles, May 1998 (available online).
Brian Hill, 'A Spiritual Diarist: John Rutty, M.D. 1698–1775)', *The Practitioner*, 187 (1961), pp. 219–23.
Eoin Magennis, '"A Land of Milk and Honey": the Physio-Historical Society, Improvement and the Surveys of Mid-Eighteenth Century Ireland', *Proceedings of the Royal Irish Academy*, 102C:6 (2002), pp. 204, 206.
John D. Post, *Food Shortage, Climatic Variability, and Epidemic Disease in Preindustrial Europe. The Mortality Peak in the early 1740s* (Ithaka: Cornell University Press, 1985).

William Harty, *An Historic Sketch of the Causes, Progress, Extent, and Mortality of the Contagious Fever Epidemic in Ireland during the Years 1817, 1818, and 1819* (1820)

Primary:
Francis Barker and John Cheyne, *An Account of the Rise, Progress, and Decline of the Fever lately Epidemical in Ireland, together*

with Communications from Physicians in the Provinces, and various Official Documents (2 vols, Dublin: Hodges and M'Arthur, 1821) (see this set, Volumes III and IV).

William Harty, *An Historic Sketch of the Causes, Progress, Extent, and Mortality of the Contagious Fever Epidemic in Ireland during the Years 1817, 1818, and 1819; with numerous Tables, Official Documents, and Private Communications, illustrative of its General History and of the System of Management adopted for its Suppression* (Dublin: Hodges and M'Arthur, 1820).

John Huxham, *Observationes de Aere, et Morbis epidemicis, ab anno 1728 ad finem anni 1737 Plymuthi factæ. His accedit opusculum de Morbo colico Damnoniensi* (London: S. Austen, 1739);

John Huxham, *Observations on the Air, and Epidemic Diseases from the Beginning of the Year 1738 to the End of the Year 1748* (translated from the Latin, London: J. Hinton, 1759–67).

Maurice O'Connell, *Morborum acutorum, et chronicorum quorundam, observationes medicinales experimentales* (Dublin: S. Powell, 1746).

John Rutty, *A Chronological History of the Weather and Seasons, and of the Prevailing Diseases in Dublin: with the various Periods, Successions, and Revolutions, during the Space of Forty Years* ... (London: Robinson and Roberts, 1770) (this volume, pp. 19–412).

Secondary:

K.H. Connell, *The Population of Ireland 1750–1845* (Oxford: Clarendon Press, 1950).

David Dickson, 'The Gap in Famines: A Useful Myth?' in E. Margaret Crawford (ed.), *Famine: The Irish Experience 900–1900* (Edinburgh: J. Donald, 1989), pp. 96–111.

David Dickson, *Arctic Ireland. The Extraordinary Story of the Great Frost and Forgotten Famine of 1740–41* (Belfast: White Row Press, 1997).

Laurence M. Geary, *Medicine and Charity in Ireland 1718–1851* (Dublin: University College Dublin Press, 2004).

Laurence M. Geary, 'Harty, William (1781–1854)', *Oxford Dictionary of National Biography* (Oxford: Oxford University Press, 2004).

J.D. Post, *Food Shortage, Climatic Variability, and Epidemic Disease in Preindustrial Europe. The Mortality Peak in the Early 1740s* (Ithaca and London: Cornell University Press, 1985).

J.D. Post, *The Last Great Subsistence Crisis of the Western World* (Baltimore: Johns Hopkins University Press, 1977).

Notes

[Jonathan Swift], *A Short View of the State of Ireland* (1727–8)

p. 3: 'Printed by S. HARDING': Sarah Harding, widow of John Harding (d. 1725) who printed five of the seven letters of the *Drapier's letters* in 1724.

p. 8, ll. 7–12: *The Thirteenth, is, where ... Nations*: reference to the Wood's halfpence controversy. In 1722 William Wood, a Wolverhampton iron master obtained a licence via the King's mistress to coin copper halfpence and farthings for circulation in Ireland. The licence caused outrage in Ireland.

p. 9, ll. 29–30: *a million of Discouragements*: a reference especially to the Cattle Acts of 1666 and 1680 (18 Chas. II, c. 2; 32 Chas. II, c. 2) that prohibited the export of live cattle to England and the Woollen Act of 1699 (10 & 11 Will III, c. 10) prohibiting the export of woollen cloth to places outside the British Isles.

p. 10, l. 20–3: *an Act of Navigation ... a thousand other unexampled Circumstances*: references to a body of legislation, the so-called commercial restraints, whereby the British parliament placed restrictions on Irish commerce.

p. 10, ll. 29–30: *L — C — J — W —'s Ghost* [Lord Chief Justice Whitshed's Ghost]: William Whitshed (1679–1727), Lord Chief Justice of the King's Bench 1714–27. Attempted unsuccessfully to have printers of several of Swift's pamphlets convicted of seditious libel. He was suspected of tricking a family connection out of an inheritance, hence the betrayal of the family motto.

p. 11, ll. 17–18: *the manner of the* Scythians: nomadic tribe of Iranian origin whose economy was based on grazing. There was a popular but misguided belief that the Irish were descended from the Sythians.

p. 12, ll. 1–2: *One third part of the Rents of* Ireland *is spent in* England: Complaints about the remittance of rents to landlords living in England grew in 1725–8 when harvests failures led to rising corn imports and concerns about the deteriorating balance of trade.

p. 12, ll. 24–5: *a sort of Silk Plad*: possibly poplin, a cotton cloth, although at the time Dublin possessed a considerable silk industry.

p. 13, ll. 11–13: ... *except the Linnen of the* North *a Trade casual corrupted and at Mercy, and some Butter from* Cork: The manufacture of linen yarn and cloth was expanding especially in Ulster and became very important after 1730; 'at mercy' is a reference to the commercial restraints that generally worked in favour of Irish linen. Cork was becoming a major centre of a butter (and meat) export trade.

p. 13, l. 18: *Let the worthy C——rs* [Commissioners]: the revenue commissioners excise and customs.

p. 14, l. 22–4: *The Families of Farmers, who pay great Rents, living in Filth and Nastiness upon Butter-milk and Potatoes* ...: a hyperbolic statement of the importance of buttermilk and potatoes in diets; they became more important as the century progressed. The failure of the grain harvests in 1725–7 forced many people to rely on potatoes and to lift the crop early.

p. 17, ll. 2–3: ... when the Hen is starved to Death, there will be no more Golden Eggs: a fear that an adverse balance of payments would ultimately drain all specie from the country.

p. 17, l. 12: *I have known an Hospital*: possibly the Dublin Foundling Hospital.

John Rutty, *A Chronological History of the Weather and Seasons, and of the Prevailing Diseases in Dublin* (1770)

p. 27, l. 21: *Thompson on the Seasons*: James Thomson, poet, *The Seasons* (London: A. Millar, 1744).

p. 28, l. 5: *Wintringham, Huxham*: Clifton Wintringham, *A Treatise of Endemic Diseases, wherein the Different Nature of Airs, Situations, Soils, Waters, Diet, &c. are mechanically Explain'd and Accounted for* (York: Grace White, 1718); *An Enquiry into the Exility of the Vessels of the Human Body, wherein Animal Identity is Explained, and Shewn Incommunicable to any Individual throughout the Whole Species* (London: Thomas Osborne, 1743); *An Essay on Contagious Diseases: more particularly on the Small-Pox, Measles, Putrid, Malignant, and Pestilential Fevers* (York: Charles Bourne, 1721). John Huxham, *An Essay on Fevers and their Various Kinds, as depending on different Constitutions of the Blood: with Dissertations on Slow Nervous Fevers; on Putrid, Pestilential, Spotted Fevers; on the Small-Pox; and on Pleurisies and Peripneumonies* (London: S. Austen, 1750); *A Dissertation on the Malignant, Ulcerous Sore-Throat* (London: J. Hinton, 1757); *An Essay on Fevers. To which is now added a Dissertation on the Malignant, Ulcerous Sore-Throat* (London: J. Hinton, 1764).

p. 28, l. 6: *Dr. Short*: Thomas Short, *A General Chronological History of the Weather, Seasons, Meteors, etc. ...* (2 vols, London: T. Longman and A. Millar, 1749).

p. 32, ll. 18–19: *Paulus Ægineta*: *De compositione medicaminum generalium ex Paulo Ægineta*, in C. Cesner, *Apparatus et delectus simplicium medicamentorum, etc.* ([Lyon?]: 1542).

p. 32, ll. 18–19: Dies ... quartus: 'The seventh and the fourteenth are the best critical days' (translation).

p. 32, l. 20: *Fernelius*: Joannes Fernelius, *A Treatise of the principall Diseases of the Eyes, gathered out of Fernelius*, in Walter Bailey, *Two Treatises, etc. Two Treatises Concerning the Preservation of Eie-Sight* (Oxford [i.e. London]: Joseph Barnes, 1616).

p. 33, ll. 1–3: Continuam ..., solvit: 'Continuous fever disperses in a second or ... third week' (translation).

p. 34, l. 18: *Dr. Fothergill*: John Fothergill, *An Account of the Sore Throat attended with Ulcers: A Disease which hath of Late Years Appeared in this City, and in Several Parts of the Nation* (London: C. Davis, 1748).

p. 38, l. 18: *Dr. Mead*: Richard Mead, *Monita et præcepta medica* (Hamburg: Grund and Holle, 1752).

p. 40, l. 8: *Dr. Rogers*: Joseph Rogers, *An Essay On Epidemic Diseases* (Dublin: W. Smith, 1734).

p. 40, l. 21: *Boate's Natural History*: Gerard Boate, *Irelands Naturall History ..., written by Gerard Boate and now published by Samuell Hartlib ... for the Common Good of Ireland ...* (London: John Wright, 1652).

p. 42, l. 1: *Bontius*: Jacobus Bontius (Jakob de Bondt), *An Account of the Diseases, Natural History, and Medicines of the East Indies, translated from the Latin. To which are added annotations by a Physician* (London: T. Noteman, 1769).

p. 42, ll. 2–11: Plerumque ... depascitur: 'Diseases generally attack mortals with such madness that they immediately dislodge them as though astonished from their mental reasoning and snatch the sick from life often within a very few days, or sometimes hours, with frenzy and continuous delirium: there are present eternal wakefulness, vomit of different colour, in particular the colour of green and rusty bile. External features grow stiff: an internal heat with huge thirst feeds upon the vital and natural faculties' (translation).

p. 42, l. 12: *Prosper Alpinus*: *Prosperi Alpini De medicina Ægyptiorum libri quatuor, etc.* (Venice, 1591).

p. 43, l. 18: *Cleghorn's Observations ...*: George Cleghorn, *Observations on the Epidemical Diseases in Minorca from the year 1744 to 1749.*

To which is prefixed, a Short Account of the Climate, Productions, Inhabitants, and Endemial Distempers of that Island (London: D. Wilson, 1751).

p. 44, l. 22: *Towne*: Richard Towne, *A Treatise of the Diseases most frequent in the West Indies, and herein more particularly of those which occur in Barbadoes* (London: J. Clarke, 1726).

p. 45, ll. 4–6: Cum anni ... judicii: 'When the season of the year has its own temperature diseases are constant and diagnoses are the best' (translation).

p. 45, l. 16 to p. 47, l. 16: Quod hyems ... syderationes: 'Because the winter fills the body with phlegm ... men both spit out and wipe their noses in the most phlegmatic winter, and tumors become loose and very white, especially in this season, and likewise other phlegmatic diseases.

In the spring the blood increases.

In the spring and summer men are greatly seized with dysentery, and blood flows from their very nostrils. But in the summer the blood still has strength and bile is raised up in the body, and this extends forth right up until autumn. But in autumn the blood becomes moderate: for bile takes possession throughout summer and autumn; something which you can recognise from the fact that men of their own accord vomit out bile at this time and in the purging of the medications very bilious things are purged: it becomes clear both from the fevers and the temperatures of men.

Black bile is both very great and very strong in autumn ....

Indeed all diseases occur in all seasons; however in certain seasons some are both increased and exacerbated. For in spring insanity and black bile and epilepsy, flowing of blood and angina and catarrh and hoarseness and coughing and leprosy and skin disease and psoriasis and very many ulcerous spots and swellings and arthritis.

But in the summer some of these: continuous fevers, and blazing heat, and vomiting recurring every three or four days, and diarrhoea and inflammation of the eyes and ear-ache and mouth ulcers and putrefaction of the private parts and sweaty beasts. But in the autumn vagrant fevers every four days and diseases of the spleen and dropsy and decay and a trickling of urine and lightness of the intestines and dysentery and diseases of the hip-bone and angina and breathlessness and dizziness and epilepsy and insanity and black bile.

But in winter pleurisy, inflammation of the lungs, and catarrh, hoarseness, coughing, chest-pains, pains of the sides and loins, headaches, vertigo, paralysis' (translations.

p. 49, l. 18: *PRIOR*: Matthew Prior (1664–1721), poet, politician and diplomat. As ambassador to Paris he negotiated the Treaty of Utrecht of 1713, popularly known as 'Matt's Peace'. Subsequently impeached and imprisoned. On release, his poems were published in 1717 with the help of Lord Harley.

p. 50, l. 22: *Dr. Pringle*: Sir John Pringle, *Observations on the Diseases of the Army in Camp and Garrison* (4th edition, London: 1764).

p. 51, l. 23: *Celsus*: Platonist writer who lived towards the end of the second century (AD).

p. 52, l. 24: *Sanctorius*: An Italian physician who in 1614 made the first recorded measurements of changes in weight, pulse and temperature taken from his own body using a primitive thermometer.

p. 53, ll. 3–6: Adiapneustia quæ ... hyeme: 'Adiapneustia (defective perspiration), which can produce malignant disease in summer but causes very little change in winter, for bodies are full of keener perspiration in summer than in winter' (translation).

p. 54. l. 10: *bill of mortality*: weekly records of deaths in Dublin.

p. 59, l. 5: *Dunkirk fever*: probably the fever at the siege of Dunkirk (1658) among the Anglo-French army.

p. 60, l. 11: *Piso*: Gulielmus Piso, *Pisonis ... de Indiæ utriusque Re Naturali et Medica libri quatuordecim ....* (Amsterdam: Elsevier, 1658).

p. 63, l. 2: *Bryan Robinson*: Bryan Robinson, *Observations on the Virtues and Operations of Medicines* (Dublin: 1752).

p. 65, l. 20: *Boyle Godfrey*: Boyle Godfrey, *A Treasure of Useful Discoveries. In two parts. I. Remarks on Divers Aliments or Eatables ... II. A Number of Valuable Discoveries of Universal Benefit to the Publick* (Dublin: 1746).

p. 67, l. 5: *Tabor*: Probably John Tabor, *Exercitationes medicæ, quæ, tam morborum quam symptomatum, in plerisque morbis rationem illustrant* (London: Guilielmi & Johannis Innys, 1724).

p. 71, l. 25: *Langrish*: Browne Langrish, *The Modern Theory and Practice of Physic: wherein the Antecedent Causes of Diseases, the Rise of the most usual Symptoms incident to them, and the true Methods of Cure, are explained according to the established Laws of Nature, and those of the Animal Oeconomy: together with a Chemical Analysis of the Urine and a Statical Examination of the Blood, in every Stage of each Distemper where Blood could be drawn with Safety* (London: A. Bettesworth and C. Hitch, 1735).

p. 74, l. 7: *exanthematous fevers*: fevers accompanied by a skin rash.

p. 75, l. 4: *petechial*: spotty.

p. 83, l. 1: *salutiserous*: beneficial, health-giving.

p. 88, l. 22: *primæ viæ*: the bowels.

p. 95, l. 22: *Doctors Rogers and Connel*: Dr Joseph Rogers, *An Essay On Epidemic Diseases: and more particularly on the Endemial Epidemics of the City of Cork, such as Fevers and Small-Pox, but more professedly on the Endemial Epidemic Fever of the Year MDCCXXXI, with an Attempt to account for the General and Special Causes producing the Same: also, the Method of Cure found most successful: in two Parts* (Dublin: S. Powell, 1734). Dr Connell, possibly Dr Maurice O'Connell (see below, p. 159).

p. 103, l. 23: Sudor Anglicus: the English sweating sickness, characterised by heavy sweats, prostration and a high fatality rate.

p. 111, ll. 1–2: *German Ephemerides*: possibly *Academiæ Cæsareo-Leopoldinæ ... Ephemerides; sive, observationum medico-physicarum a celeberrimis viris ... communicatarum* (5 vols, Frankfurt: 1712–22).

p. 118, ll. 21–3: *Omnes fructus ... intereunt*: 'All seasonal fruits are bitter and unripe, scarcely do you hear the cicada, butterflies rarely fly about, many song birds die amid the casting of their feathers' (translation).

p. 123, ll. 23–4: *decoctum album*: a medicine probably containing mistletoe (*Viscum album*).

p. 123, l. 24: *testacea*: a species of sedge.

p. 124, l. 1: *diascordium*: a mixture or treacle of plants etc, including roses, liquorice, spikenard, myrrh, horehound (a plant of the mint family), pepper, valerian, gentian, St John's wort, *etc.*

p. 124, ll. 15–17: *Assiduis imbribus ... &c*: 'With constant showers diseases generally become long fevers, flowings of the belly, putrefactions, prolapse of the cartilage, [and] ensiformis etc.' (translation) [in botany 'ensiformis' refers to a sword-shaped, pointed leaf. The sense here is uncertain].

p. 129, l. 21: *Baglivi*: Nicolas Andry De Bois-Regard, *An Account of the Breeding of Worms in Human Bodies their Nature and Several Sorts: their Effects, Symptoms, and Prognosis: with the True Means to avoid them, and Medicines to cure them: with Letters to the Author on this Subject from M. Nicolas Hartsoeker at Amsterdam and M. George Baglivi at Rome* (London: s.n., 1701).

p. 129, l. 22: *cantharides*: Spanish fly, a preparation of dried blister beetles.

p. 133, l. 1: *peripneumonia notha*: a severe form of pneumonia.

p. 134, l. 10: *dog-days*: the hottest period of the year.

p. 135, l. 13: *chin-coughs*: whooping cough.

p. 146, l. 12: *miliary fevers*: spotted fevers.

p. 152, l. 21: *parotids*: salivary glands.

p. 159, ll. 10–11: *Dr. Connell's Observationes Medicinales*: Maurice O'Connell, *Morborum acutorum, et chronicorum quorundam, observationes medicinales experimentales* (Dublin: S. Powell, 1746).

p. 160, l. 10: *colliquative state*: symptomatic of a wasting illness.

p. 162, ll. 14–20: *Si sicca ... nascuntur*: 'If a dry summer has had north winds and if a dry autumn has also been breathed upon by the same north winds, good health befalls all softer bodies (e.g. women), but dry inflammation of the eyes, and fevers, sometimes acute, sometimes long, and those diseases which are born from black bile, can press upon harder things' (translation).

p. 165, l. 6: *Sydenham*: Thomas Sydenham, *Observationes medicae circa morborum acutorum historiam et curationem* ... (London: Gualteri Kettilby, 1676).

p. 165, l. 14: *Dr. Berkley*: George Berkeley, Bishop of Cloyne, *Siris: A Chain of Philosophical Reflexions and Inquiries concerning the Virtues of Tar Water: and Divers other Subjects connected together and arising one from another* (London: W. Innys, C. Hitch and C. Davis, 1744).

p. 172, l. 22: *Forestus*: possibly Petrus Forestus, *Specimina individualia ... cognationis seu dependentiæ morborum ex P. F. operibus ... collecta* in Johann Samuel Carl and Johann Jacob Schlierbach, *Johannis Samuelis Carl Historia medica pathologico-therapeutica: in qva morborum circumstantiae perpepetuae [sic] essentiales & extra-essentiales aphoristice expenduntur* (Hafniae: Impensis Iacobi Prevssii, 1738).

p. 176, l. 19: *Melite*: Malta.

p. 183, l. 6: *aspera arteria*: the windpipe.

p. 185, l. 3: *bolus of theriaca andromachi*: a pill or compound (sometimes containing poppy juice) used as an antidote to poison.

p. 185, l. 8: *Tournefort*: Joseph Pitton De Tournefort, *A Voyage into the Levant: ... to which is prefix'd the author's life; ... as also his eulogium, pronounc'd by M. Fontenelle* ... (3 vols, London: D. Midwinter, 1741).

p. 186, ll. 5–6: *angina maligna* ...: angina is a tightening ('strangulation'), today usually used to describe chest pains but in the past also to sore throats etc.

p. 186, l. 14: *deglutition*: swallowing.

p. 188: l. 14: *antiphlogistic*: anti inflammatory.

p. 188, l. 18: *alexipharmic*: antidote to poison.

p. 189, l. 24: *sanious*: a discharge of serum.

p. 190, l. 17: *Dr. Home*: Francis Home, *An Inquiry into the Nature, Cause, and Cure of the Croup* (Edinburgh: A. Kincaid and J. Bell, 1765).

p. 195, l. 8: *lentor*: slowness, sluggishness.

p. 202, l. 23: *mock-suns*: Parhelions: bright spots in the sky on either side of the sun caused by refraction.

p. 208, ll. 21–2: *membrana Schneideri*: mucous membrane lining the nasal cavity.

p. 225, ll. 19–20: *lord Anson*: the vessel, Lord Anson, voyaged around the world in 1750–2.

p. 244, l. 17: *tabid*: emaciated wasted, consumptive.

p. 261, l. 16: *hemiplegias*: paralysis of one side of the body.

p. 265, l. 8: *hectics*: recurrent fever typically accompanying tuberculosis.

p. 287, l. 5: *COR.*: corollaries.

p. 294, l. 5: *putrid, inflammatory*: inflammatory fevers include chicken pox, erypsipelas and smallpox; putrid fevers include itch and scabbiness, catarrh.

p. 295, ll. 13–14: *Hippocrates's Epidemics*: In his book *On Epidemics*, Hippocrates advised doctors to note daily specific symptoms of what they observed in order to discover the natural history of an illness.

p. 296, l. 7: *Galen*: Claudius Galen (AD 131–201). Compiler and systemizer of Greco-Roman medicine, physiology, pharmacy and anatomy; his ideas dominated medical thinking for 1500 years.

p. 298, ll. 9–16: C*ontinuam febrem … profectam*: 'A second or (for something which is very slow) a third week disperses continuous fever. If any continuous fever stretches beyond the second day, regard this as a symptom originating either from inner phlegm or its departure or from putrefaction that has infected the insides' (translation).

p. 298, l. 24: *Le Clerc*: Daniel Le Clerc, *Histoire de la Medecine* … (Nouvelle edition, Amsterdam: 1723).

p. 306, l. 8: *the venæ bibulæ*: 'drinking veins' – i.e. pores on the skin.

p. 308, l. 15: *the divine old man*: Thomas Sydenham, *Epistolæ responsoriæ duæ, prima de morbis epidemicis ab anno 1675 ad annum 1680* (London: Walter Kettilby, 1680).

p. 310, l. 4: *the New Stile*: Ireland switched to the Gregorian calendar (New Style) on 2 September 1752.

p. 312, l. 16: *the king's infirmary*: probably the King's Hospital School (the Blue Coat Hospital).

p. 331, l. 10: *fauces*: the opening at the back of the mouth.

p. 338, l. 6: *subsultus*: a convulsive movement.

p. 348, ll. 8–9: *cortex Peruvianus*: Cinchona bark.

p. 374, ll. 3–4: *hœmoptoes*: haemoptysis – the coughing up of blood.

p. 376, l. 4: *tenesmus*: continual wish to evacuate the bowels.

p. 399, l. 10: *in another work*: Possibly Thomas Short, *A General Chronological History of the Weather, Seasons, Meteors, etc. ...* (2 vols, London: T. Longman and A. Millar, 1749).

p. 407, l. 17: *depuration*: purification; cleansing (of infections, etc.).

p. 409, ll. 1–2: *Ægineta* ... decimus-quartus: 'The seventh and the fourteenth are the best critical days' (translation).

William Harty, *An Historic Sketch of the Causes, Progress, Extent, and Mortality of the Contagious Fever Epidemic in Ireland during the Years 1817, 1818, and 1819* (1820)

p. 418, l. 13: *Dr. Rogers of Cork*: Dr Joseph Rogers, *An Essay On Epidemic Diseases* (Dublin: W. Smith 1734).

p. 419, l. 11: *O'Connell and Rutty*: Maurice O'Connell, *Morborum acutorum, et chronicorum quorundam, observationes medicinales experimentales* (Dublin: S. Powell, 1746); John Rutty, *A Chronological History of the Weather and Seasons, and of the Prevailing Diseases in Dublin: with the various Periods, Successions, and Revolutions, during the Space of Forty Years ...* (London: Robinson and Roberts, 1770) (this volume, pp. 19–412)

p. 419, l. 21: *Boate*: Gerard Boate, *Irelands Naturall History ..., written by Gerard Boate and now published by Samuell Hartlib ... for the Common Good of Ireland ...* (London: John Wright, 1652).

p. 420, l. 6: *Dr. Barker*: Dr Francis Barker (*c*.1771–1859). Professor of Chemistry, Trinity College, Dublin; physician to the Cork Street Fever Hospital, Dublin. Author (with John Cheyne) of *An Account of the Rise, Progress, and Decline of the Fever lately Epidemical in Ireland, together with Communications from Physicians in the Provinces, and various Official Documents* (2 vols, Dublin: Hodges and M'Arthur, 1821) (see this set, Volumes III and IV).

p. 420, l. 26: *Dr. Murray of Cavan*: his 'Account of the Epidemic Fever as it appeared in Cavan' appears in Barker and Cheyne.

p. 420, l. 35: *'Typhus gravior of Cullen'*: probably a reference to the classification of diseases by William Cullen (1710–90), professor of the

Practice of Physic at the University of Edinburgh. He wrote *Genera morborum* containing the *Synopsis nosologiae methodicae*, translated and published as *A Methodical System of Nosology* (Stockbridge, MA: Cornelius Sturtevant, 1808).

p. 421, l. 2: *Dr. Cheyne*: John Cheyne (1777–1836), Physician General to the army in Ireland. Co-author with Francis Barker (see above).

p. 421, l. 13: *Dr. Crampton*: Sir Philip Crampton (1777–1858), Dublin physician. Surgeon to the Meath Hospital, Dublin 1798–1858 and the Westmoreland Lock Hospital, 1806. Surgeon-General 1813. President of the Royal College of Surgeons in Ireland on four occasions.

p. 421, l. 19: *Dr. Clarke*: Dr James Clarke, a contributor to Barker and Cheyne, where his early death is regretted.

p. 424, ll. 6–7: *Smith's Kerry*: Charles Smith, *The Antient and Present State of the County of Kerry …* (Dublin: 1756).

p. 424, ll. 9–10: *General Chronological History of the weather*: Rutty's, *A Chronological History of the Weather and Seasons.*

p. 424, ll. 30–4 to p. 425, ll. 18–22: *Ab horrendo hoc et infando sicco gelu … gelu penitùs putrescebant*: 'From this most dreadful and unutterable dry chill there arose not only a great slaughter of all beasts, but also a lamentable pestilence that destroyed all sort of plants and vegetables. The very birds of the sky and other animals adapted to human diet perished in great numbers on account of the intense stiffness of the cold season; and – something which still increased much more seriously the mass of deadly evils – those swelling roots (commonly called potatoes), generally a constant and wholesome source of nourishment for the common people and inferior habitants of this kingdom, became utterly rotten from this most dreadful and lengthy chill' (translation).

p. 425, l. 27: *Huxham's account*: John Huxham, *Observationes de Aere, et Morbis epidemicis, ab anno 1728 ad finem anni 1737 Plymuthi factœ. His accedit opusculum de Morbo colico Damnoniensi* (London: S. Austen, 1739); *Observations on the Air, and Epidemic Diseases from the Beginning of the Year 1738 to the End of the Year 1748* (translated from the Latin, London: J. Hinton, 1759–67).

p. 425, ll. 28–35. *Adeo sævum regnabat … fere simus vitales*: 'Cold reigned over the age to such an extent that all kinds of wine when left exposed outside soon congealed; indeed so did the sea itself by the shore, something which happens here at any rate most rarely. Countless plants and trees perish, as does even the plant broom itself; hardly could you see a green blade of grass. Whatever has been exposed to the air freezes swifter than words – and stiffening with cold even in our beds alongside glowing fires, we are so sluggish on account of the dreadful cold that generally we are scarcely alive' (translation).

p. 426, ll. 14–18: *Verbo dicam ... frequentissimè ventilatum fuit*: 'The whole aforementioned two-year period, experiencing that very cold winter, was steeped in scattered showers, and was very frequently fanned by eastern and northern blasts beyond the usual custom of the island' (translation).

p. 426, ll. 24–7: *Major fortè nunquam ... fumosa quasi apparet*: 'Never by chance has a greater dryness been observed: springs immediately become dry and rivers dry up. Even though all types of hygroscopes designate an extremely dry temperature of the air, nonetheless the whole atmosphere appears very dense and, as it were, smoky' (translation).

p. 426, ll. 29–31: ... *perpetuæ fere decidunt ... corruptum, et fructus prorsus fatui*: '... generally perpetual showers fall and everything flows with excessive humidity; whence the harvest is completely unfruitful, the corn almost corrupt and fruit thoroughly tasteless' (translation).

p. 426, ll. 32–4: ... *torrida valde et aridissima ... frumentum optimum*: 'A very parched and very dry temperature burnt almost everything: hence a ripe and fertile harvest, excellent corn' (translation).

p. 428, ll. 29–32 to p. 429, ll. 30–2: *Tussis vehemens ... crescit magnitudinem*: 'Violent coughing with suffocating angina and fever destroyed many horses; indeed even the breed of oxen is often snatched away by such a condition. The wool-bearing flock labours greatly under thinness and dry coughing; countless sheep perish, all of whose liver greatly swells and becomes hard; but the bladder swollen with black bile increases to huge magnitude' (translation).

p. 430, ll. 5–10: *Hinc ... cadaveribus conflata*: 'From this (i.e. from the chill) a deadly dearth of crop and a dreadful famine raging savagely among the poor and the lower classes; hence the common people's sources of nourishment as a consequence of those perverse and corrupt roots (potatoes) were mingled with vegetables of corrupt juices and with the corpses of diseased animals' (translation).

p. 430, ll. 20–2: ... *quæ sensim ... hyemen stragem edidit*: '...which, augmenting sensation through the whole autumn, produced a great and unbelievable slaughter throughout the following winter' (translation).

p. 431, ll. 24–5: *Groans of Ireland*: Anon, *The Groans of Ireland: in a Letter to a Member of Parliament* (Dublin: G. Faulkner, 1741).

p. 433, ll. 29–32: *Præcedunt aliquando ... magnâ virium et spirituum dissipatione*: 'Sometimes stiffness and shuddering advance with heat, as happens in fevers; as it follows, the sick man grows feverish with his tongue white at the beginning, but as the disease progresses, more often and often dry, and at some time or another black, with the great dissipation of strength and of breath' (translation).

p. 433, ll. 34–5: *Contagium ab effluviis ... manantibus ortum*: 'The infection arose from flowings out of the diseased body or from its excrements exuding' (translation).

p. 434, ll. 3–8: *Exeunte Augusto ... epidemicè grassabatur*: 'As August departed there came into sight a certain continuous epidemic fever, which raged savagely in certain places through the whole autumn among the lower classes in particular and by attacking many, it proceeded in epidemic fashion right up until or around the winter solstice' (translation).

p. 434, ll. 10–24: ... *febris hæc dysenteriæ ... invasit et adveniente hyeme penitus disparuit*: 'This recent fever now gave way to dysentery that increased with renewed strength until the chill at last being dissolved and with the arrival by a favourable change of a dry and northern spring, the same fever sprouted again, and spreading far and wide it consumed almost the whole population indiscriminately: rejoicing in the predominance of dysentery and all other epidemics at the same time, and since it was spread about with excessive heat from the arrival of the summer, in the same progression among the people it lasted roughly until the end of August: from which time gradually retreating, it did not disappear in the following winter, but in the spring of the year 1742, just as also in the following summer, the aforesaid continuous fever returned but in comparison to the preceding year, it attacked fewer people and utterly disappeared with the arrival of winter' (translation).

p. 434, ll. 27–34: *Dysenteria cruenta frequens; Dysenteria plures cruciat; ... febres malignæ jam nec vi, nec numero adeo sæviunt; ... grassatur* adhuc *febris ... ,sæva dysenteria consumit; ... jam maxime furit febris pestilentialis ... saltem excedunt solitum numerum.*: 'a frequent and bloody dysentery'; 'Dysentery tortures many'; ... 'malignant fevers do not rage so severely either in terms of strength or number'; '...malignant scurvy [i.e. *febris nautica*, a fever among sailors] still proceeds and kills many; and not infrequently savage dysentery consumes those whom the fever had almost left'; '...now a pestilential fever rages greatly and sends very many to the underworld; certainly deaths now exceed their customary number by at least six times' (translations).

p. 435, ll. 19–25: ... *jam grassatur febris ... popellum multos; Ineunte vere (anni 1740) ... hinc in vulgum quòque* sparsa *maximam edidit stragem*: '...now a putrefying spotted fever proceeds, which sends very many sailors and many among the populace to the underworld'. 'At the beginning of spring (1740) two war ships were brought to this harbour [Plymouth]; from these more than two hundred sick were instantly put to land, and the majority of these laboured under a malignant or rather pestilential fever; spreading hence among the people also, it caused the greatest slaughter' (translations).

p. 435, ll. 26–7: ... *inter nautas verò præcipuè et maximè in nosocomiis*: '... but in particular among sailors and very great in regard to nosocomial infection' (translation) [A nosocomial infection is a disease originating in hospital; the passage here refers to the spread of infection from ships to the general population].

p. 435, ll. 29–32: ... *sedulo inquirens has (febres) ... morbi seminium*: '... zealously investigating these fevers I find that generally there is a contagious spreading of scurvy, indeed when one or two convalescing sailors approaches those regions, it is not safe to receive those recuperating from the contagious fever: the origin of the disease still clings for long to the clothes' (translation).

p. 437, ll. 24–5: ... *another Committee was also appointed*: 'Report of a Select Committee Appointed to Examine the State of Contagious Fever in the Metropolis, and into the Conditions of the Institutions for the Care and Prevention of the Same', *British Parliamentary Papers, 1818* (332), vol. VII.

p. 440, ll. 8–13: *Efflorescentia fuit ... hoc morbo symptoma*: 'There was as it were a blossoming of measles in the trunk of the body and in the limbs: in some, little red spots emulating the blossoming of measles; in others purple, but in some yellow and black. Profuse haemorrhaging from the nostrils is a very common symptom in this disease' (translation).

p. 440, ll. 20–1: ... *dolores rheumatismum nonnunquam aut lumbaginem æmulantes*: '...rheumatic pains or sometimes pains emulating lumbago' (translation).

p. 440, l. 28 to p. 441, ll. 24–6: *Hinc denique luctuosa et terribilis: ... observatum noverim*: 'Hence finally a mournful and terrible slaughter of men, which in terms of the number of the dead is thought not only to equal but also to transcend the very plague itself which once proceeded in this region. With the years 1740 and 1741 I myself believe that a minimum of 80,000 sick men perished on the occasion of the aforesaid disasters, and I know that this was observed by many extremely sharp-sighted men paying serious attention to this fatal event' (translation).

p. 442, l. 15 to p. 444, l. 5: ... *hinc complurium* ... aeris constitutio: '... hence the fodder of very many acute and deadly diseases; at that time the epidemic condition of the air greatly favoured the spreading and extending of these far and wide' (translation).

p. 444, l. 18: *Dr. Bracken*: his 'Medical Report of the Fever Hospital of Waterford' was included in Barker and Cheyne.

p. 446, l. 17 to. p. 448, l. 5: ... *quamvis enim febrem ... feleciter cessisse*: '... for even though I do not doubt that this fever was of the inflammatory kind, having learned from repeated experience, I am certain that a phlebotomy, which was very frequently repeated so that the sole cause, namely, inflammation, of this bloody fever might be removed en masse, did not happen so successfully' (translation).

p. 448, ll. 9–11: ... *nec alia quoque ... reprimere valeant*: '... and no other anti-inflammatory method has the power to check the terrible frenzy that arrives with this fever or the tenacious wakefulness' (translation).

p. 448, l. 13: *alvine evacuation*: purging.

p. 448, ll. 20–1: ...*peculiaris cujusdam inflammationis fuisse participem*: '... was a participant in a certain peculiar inflammation' (translation).

p. 448, l. 23 – p. 450, l. 5: ... *experientiâ quotidianâ ..., frequentèr evaserunt*: 'It is evident from daily practice that the sick raging on account of a frenetic madness, who got up naked from their beds against the will of their nurses, and exposed themselves to the freer air (receiving no harm whatsoever from this) were by this fortuitous chance nonetheless alleviated in no small degree from that terrible madness ... Even the poor lying down under the same fever became mad, with a more liberal drinking of common water and without even the slightest form of regulation or preparation of remedy, were freed from the madness and frequently escaped' (translation).

p. 450, l. 7: *acescent*: sour.

p. 451, l. 25: *Dr. Barry*: Dr Milner Barry, contributed 'Observations on the Medical Topography of Cork, as Connected with the Late Epidemic Fever' to Barker and Cheyne.

p. 454, l. 21: *Dr. Percival*: probably Dr Edward Percival (or Perceval), sometime editor of the *Dublin Hospital Reports*, a Dublin medical journal. There was also Dr Robert Perceval who was one of the fourteen original members of the General Board of Health, formed in March 1820.

Index

For Product Safety Concerns and Information please contact our EU representative GPSR@taylorandfrancis.com
Taylor & Francis Verlag GmbH, Kaufingerstraße 24, 80331 München, Germany

www.ingramcontent.com/pod-product-compliance
Ingram Content Group UK Ltd.
Pitfield, Milton Keynes, MK11 3LW, UK
UKHW020025200926
475702UK00014B/2056
* 9 7 8 1 1 3 8 1 1 1 4 6 2 *